The Prostate Cancer Primer

The Prostate Cancer Primer

✦

It's Not A Disease Just for Older Men Anymore

Dr. Nicholas R. Hild, PhD. Professor,

College of Technology and Applied Sciences

Arizona State University

and

Dr. Patricia A. Pierce, ND

Naturopathic Consultant

with

<u>Foreword</u> *by:*

Dr. Gordon Grado, MD, Brachytherapist;

Southwest Oncology Centers

iUniverse, Inc.

New York Lincoln Shanghai

The Prostate Cancer Primer
It's Not A Disease Just for Older Men Anymore

iUniverse, Inc.

For information address:
iUniverse, Inc.
2021 Pine Lake Road, Suite 100
Lincoln, NE 68512
www.iuniverse.com

ISBN: 0-595-31125-3

Printed in the United States of America

Contents

FOREWORD

by

Dr. Gordon Grado, MD, Brachytherapist,
Southwest Oncology Centers
Scottsdale, Arizona

In the 2+ years that it has taken to complete this book, nearly 450,000 men have been diagnosed with prostate cancer! During that same period, more than 58,000 men died from prostate cancer—about the same as the number of U.S. service-men killed in the entire 10+ years of the Vietnam war. Yet the visibility of this pandemic is overshadowed by publicity and efforts to cure other types of cancers, along with diseases like AIDS and (new in 2003) SARS, that account for only a small fraction of the number of men dying from prostate cancer each and every year!

The medical community, at least that group which specializes in prostate disease, understands that the incidence of prostate cancer is increasing, and instead of being confined to older men, the age of onset is getting younger. Depending upon whose statistics you use, prostate cancer kills more than 29,000 men every year, and this year prostate cancer will be diagnosed in more than 220,000 U.S. men.

Occasionally, an event is publicized that brings prostate cancer to the forefront of medical news. These events usually make headlines for a day or two, then fade from the public's radar like stars disappearing into the rising sunlight. Unfortu-nately, what the medical community knows about prostate cancer and what the general population knows are not the same thing: a pandemic is taking place and it's time the general public was made aware.

As alarming as the magnitude of the numbers are, the fact that we are diagnosing prostate cancer in younger and younger men *at an ever-increasing rate,* should be sending a message to the general population; more research needs to be funded and more and better communication between the medical community and the population at risk needs to be accomplished or the situation will get worse.

In this book, Dr. Hild and Dr. Pierce take a different approach to communicate as much of the latest information about prostate cancer as can be presented without impediment of medical jargon as is humanly possible. To be sure, there are books that have been written which attempt to provide men with real-life stories of what treatments are available and what worked and what didn't work, but most of those quoted in references in this text (see Wentworth and O'Hara for two of the best) were first-hand accounts that are intended to teach by example. This text, on the other hand, while citing several case examples seeks to provide men who are newly diagnosed with prostate cancer as to what options for treatment there are, and more importantly, both the upside and downside of such treatments as reviewed in scientific literature.

The facts and information provided in this text are presented from an authoritative point of view because, besides being a successful research professor in his own field, Dr. Hild is also a prostate cancer victim. When he first came to see me, he had seen two nationally reputed urologists and two other brachytherapists, seeking opinions and advice about which treatment would be the best alternative for his particular cancer. During our experience together, Dr. Hild made the observation that information available to the average man faced with prostate cancer seemed at best to be convoluted, if not overwhelmingly confusing. The scientific and medical jargon in most information in the scientific literature on the subject appears to be intentionally obscure; most men would be totally confused if they tried to use it to make decisions about what they should do about their cancer treatment options.

Thus this text is not filled with charts, diagrams, drawings of prostate glands, or cancer cells. In my experience, and Dr. Hild confirms this cultural observation, *guys who have been diagnosed generally don't want to see all the anatomical and medical dialog. They don't want to talk about it; they just want an honest appraisal of their options and to get on with fixing it!*

Recently we have seen articles in the popular press, verifying what Dr. Hild and Dr. Pierce are saying. Noted Urology Department Chair, Dr. Fray Marshall at Emory University, probably said it best in a *USA Today* article (July 23, 2003)**: *"Men, on average, are not likely to lobby or be vocal about their prostate, erectile dys-*

function, urinary incontinence, loss of manhood and all the implications related to that."

Fray further noted that Hamilton Jordan, (the former Jimmy Carter aide who chronicled his battle with prostate and two other forms of cancer in a best-selling book, *No Such Thing As A Bad Day*, agrees. In the book, Jordan noted that "*Women do better than we do at this stuff because they talk about their health and they network more; it's hard to get men to do that.*"

> **(Editors Note: Available at www.usatoday.com; August 15, 2003, an *excellent* summation article of what this Primer is all about: information for men diagnosed with prostate cancer)

This text is precisely that: a discussion of options and treatments, but it's much more, because it's written at the lay-level and specifically avoids the use of medical and technical jargon which obscures the message. You won't find Anatomy 101, or even a lot of Physiology and Toxicology discussed here except as it relates to diet and nutrition in the special chapter devoted to prevention of long-term health impacts of prostate cancer.

Dr. Hild and Dr. Pierce found that most of the literature available to inquiring minds appears in places like *AARP Newsletters, The Christian Science Monitor, Redbook, Men's Health, Reader's Digest*, and *Psychology Today,* where the articles don't address the real concerns of (diagnosed) men and seem to be presented as so much milqtoast. Worse, many of those articles are written by non-scientifically-savvy writers and are misleading or sometimes just plain inaccurate. Most are exploring the psychological issues associated with prostate cancer: such things as "*success rates*" with no explanation for age of men whose rates are being quoted, no real information about what the difference is in the actual "*procedures*" (i.e. seed implants, surgery, hormones, etc.) or details of what a biopsy of the prostate gland actually *is* (i.e. how many needles are used and migration pathways that are left afterwards are not discussed), and probably most important—what "*after-effects*" (sometimes softly referred to as, "side-effects") will each treatment cause?

This last one is the subject doctors like to talk least about with patients, and knowing that men are also very reluctant to discuss such "sticky" topics, the sexual and urinary after-effects are usually handled with a hand wave and a wink, if at all.

In my many years of experience giving papers at medical conferences to other doctors and researchers in this field, I can confirm that the medical community appears to be less than forthcoming about all these subjects. Dr. Hild once told me, *"It's as though doctors receive training in 'how to conduct procedures' and let the patient deal with explanations about their physical and emotional needs by seeking psychologists or other professionals to talk to"* while some try to avoid such discussions completely by referring patients to various texts or literature.

As a doctor and brachytherapist for nearly 20 years in treating several thousand men, I can certainly confirm those observations; the medical community *has* intentionally avoided sounding the alarm! Prostate cancer needs to be prioritized for a cure at the same level as a cure for breast cancer in women is currently being funded. I'm not sure why, but the medical community has been less than forthcoming about what we know and what we don't when it comes to prostate cancer.

Dr. Patricia Pierce, who specializes in herbal and naturapathic medicine and especially in those supplements and compounds that are strongest in preventative health care, has written extensively on the role diet plays in cancer prevention. The information in this text in the nutrition chapter alone could be as important to the prostate cancer patient as the *Atkin's Diet Book* is to people trying to lose weight. But in contrast to dieters, this text is for life and death decision-making.

Thus, what is presented here is intended to send a message and a wake-up call.

Prostate Cancer rates are increasing in younger men!

The fact that most popular press publishers won't take a chance on a book that doesn't have the prospect of selling thousands of copies speaks volumes about our priorities. This is *not* fiction and it's *not* destined to be a bestseller, but there are at least 29,000 men out there this year who might reduce their risk of dying if they just follow the advice in this book:

Seek out multiple opinions on treatment for *your* specific case!

Doctors who specialize in urology and prostate disease will most likely not endorse this book; it's too honest and speaks to sensitive issues within the medical community. But they are the very professionals who should endorse this book, because its not an indictment of medical practice, after all. It's a long-overdue book of advice that should be on the waiting room tables in every urologist, oncologist, and radiologist's office as well as in every hospital and clinic where prostate cancer treatment takes place.

The alarm is being sounded and the ***Primer On Prostate Cancer*** is calling all men to respond. Buy the book, read it, then give it to all your friends to read. Almost one million men diagnosed since Y2K became an echo will tell you they wish such information had been available when they were diagnosed. Dr. Hild was one of them; his response to the alarm is this great and honest advice intended to benefit the next million men who are diagnosed. Let us hope they all get successful treatment and live long and healthy lives.

PROLOG

INTRODUCTION

LET'S START WITH THE BASICS: *What* is the Prostate Gland?

First things first: Let's learn to pronounce the word correctly. *"Pros'-tate"....*the word is *not* pronounced with an "r" following the first "t." It is *not* "Pros'trate!" That word describes the position of lying down and is not remotely related to the gland we are concerned with here, although it may be the position you envision yourself being in when the doctor tells you that your biopsy is positive. If you read this book, the chances of ending up *prostrate* from the effects of *pros-tate* cancer are very small, But you should know that incorrectly pronouncing the word in public has the same effect on the listener as running fingernails over a blackboard, so learn to pronounce the word correctly....it's *"Pros' tate"....*and only men (not women) have one!

The Healthy Cell News, (Spring 2002) describes the *prostate* as a doughnut-shaped gland that lies below a man's bladder and surrounds the urethra, the canal that carries urine and semen through the penis. Its function is to secrete fluids that lubricate the urethra and increase sperm motility. The prostate is also a muscle. It helps provide the power to expel seminal fluid through the urethra during ejaculation, and works in conjunction with the bladder muscles to control the flow of urine. It's the "pump that pulsates the flow" of seminal fluid out of the testicles sac and through the penis, so it is vitally important to a man's quality of (sex) life.

The prostate is only about as big as a peanut until a boy reaches puberty, whereupon it begins to grow to the size of a walnut and stays that size throughout young adulthood. For most men, as they enter their 40's and 50's, the prostate begins to grow again in size. It's a normal part of the aging process due to hormonal changes. This is when an enzyme called 5-alpha-reductase, commonly found in the cells of the prostate, scrotal skin, testicles and scalp, increases its activity, converting beneficial testosterone into dihdrotestosterone and causes cells to multiply excessively. This leads to prostatic enlargement, known as "Benign Prostatic Hyperplasia" (BPH) or an enlarged prostate.

But let us not worry about understanding technical or medical jargon. Let us just say that BPH has the effects on a majority of men over age 50 of increasing the frequency of urination, interrupting sleep, bladder pain, and other symptoms; even male pattern baldness is associated with BPH! But having BPH is *not*, by itself, an indication that the prostate gland is cancerous. So when your physician does a digital rectal exam (DRE) and mutters something like, "*Yep, you have an enlarged prostate…*" don't jump out the window. Most likely it's normal and benign and may or may not need treatment to relieve symptoms, but it most likely is *not* cancer.

It is when a man begins to cope with the nighttime urination frequency increase and accompanying bladder pain and/or sleep interruption that the first visit to the doctor usually occurs. Often BPH is diagnosed and, where the condition is thought to be benign, a procedure called transurethral prostatic resection (TURP) is performed. In this procedure, the abnormal tissue is cut away from the urethra and for most men, relief of the symptoms follows. A large percentage of men who have this procedure performed, however, have complications within a few months of the TURP, and the procedure often has to be repeated. Doctors think, however, that this doesn't mean that cancer of the prostate is any more (or less) likely. Continued PSA blood tests should still be ordered in routine physical exams (discussed in Chapters 1 and 2).

Not all men have BPH or symptoms that lead them to a doctor for evaluation. That is why it is critical for men over the age of 40 to have annual physical exams that include a DRE and PSA blood test. Cancer can be present and not cause any symptoms for years, so it is vital that these exams begin in early middle age.

Thus the prostate gland is a vital organ and must be kept healthy through the judicious monitoring process as a man ages. Because so little is published about the problems of prostate health, one of the missions of this book is to raise the visibility of prostate cancer and make prostate health a high priority for men of all ages. Prostate cancer is as pervasive in men as breast cancer is in women, and yet men seem to know so much less about it. Hopefully, after reading this book, that will change.

There is one thing that all men should be aware of: statistics have shown that almost 100% of men will have prostate cancer, if they live long enough. So be open-minded, get regular physical exams, and treat your prostate with the same respect and importance you do to keep your teeth healthy by having a yearly check-up.

DEFINITIONS

While we are on the subject of "definitions," there are just a few more we need to learn:

Brachytherapy: the word used to identify the process of implanting (radioactive) seeds in the treatment of cancer tumors. This technique is used to radiate tumors with "seeds" that are supplied to "brachytherapists" (i.e. doctors who specialize in radiology and oncology) for various cancer types, including breast cancer and prostate cancer.

Prostatectomy: the surgical procedure for removing the prostate gland. Also referred to as a "*radical* prostatechtomy" because the procedure eliminates the organ entirely, resulting in various side effects that may include urinary and erection dysfunction.

Thermotherapy: the process of shrinking the prostate gland or hemorrhoids with the application of heat.

Cryogenics: the process of using extreme cold to treat cancer tumors which, statistics show, may cause all the same after effects as radical prostatectomy.

MORE DEFINITIONS...

External Beam Radiation: the process of radiating the prostate gland with an externally applied radiation beam. This treatment may be used by itself or followed (or preceded) by brachytherapy. E-Beam "treatment" may also be used to ensure that, where cancer cells may have migrated outside the gland but are still in the groin area, they will be irradiated and eliminated. When used to treat cancer tumors inside the gland, it is usually done in 5-day-a-week treatments for 5 or six weeks duration. Side effects include radiation burning in the anus and colon areas that my cause bleeding and pain for a long time after treatment.

Robotic Radical Prostatechtomy: the same "process" as surgery to remove the prostate gland defined above, but with the use of robotics, sometimes referred to as the Vitti process (from Vattikuti Urology Institute, Detroit, MI) or the de Vinci system (www.goldjournal.net). This relatively new procedure reduces the side effects of prostatechtomies, although it may still result in penile nerve damage and/or sexual dysfunction.

COMMENTARY

The American Cancer Society estimates that there were 30,200 men who died of prostate cancer in 2003 (*www.cancer.org*), second only to deaths from lung and bronchus cancer. Other literature places the number of deaths at 29,000 (See Chapter 6). The NPCC (June, 2002) reported that 500 of the 30,200 (expected) prostate cancer deaths that occurred in 2002 would be in Arizona (i.e. Arizona statistics have not yet been compiled as of this writing).

A 1996 study reported in the *Journal of Clinical Cancer,* Parker, et al. showed that prostate cancer accounted for 41% of all cancers in males and a death rate of 14% for all cancers in both men and women. In the same report, breast cancer in women accounted for 31% of all cancers in women—10% less than the men's incident rate for prostate cancer—yet society is made much more aware of breast cancer (and more publicity is published about its effects) than about men's prostate cancer. Why is that?

It's been said that "*statistics lie and liars use statistics,*" so it is important not to get unnecessarily sidetracked by the numbers. We see reports and research results every day in the media which contradict and confound medical information. What is important to realize, however, is that not enough attention is being paid to prostate cancer, even where statistics continually show that something is going on. Most people believe the most prevalent forms of cancer for men and women are lung and breast cancer, respectively. According to the latest CDC survey results (2002), however, prostate cancer is by far the most prevalent cancer in men, and by a *big* margin.

Thus for men, prostate cancer is even more of a risk than the medical community would have us believe. And, the percent of *total prostate* cancers is increasing at a steeper rate than all other cancers. Some medical statistics show that this rate increase may track the statistics that show men are living longer. However, what is not appreciated, even in the medical community, is that the average age of men diagnosed with prostate cancer is declining, as younger and younger men are discovering cancer cells in their prostate glands.

As shown on Table 1, the most common cancers measured by incidences per 100,000 men in Arizona show prostate cancer is 114.4, while the next leading (lung cancer) incidence rate is 75.8 per 100,000. That's a huge difference! The CDC report shows similar data for all the other states, so it is no statistical anomaly.

Nationally, it is fairly well known that if a man lives long enough, it's almost certain he will have prostate cancer. At age 85 and above, there is a 90% probability that prostate cancer will be present; whether or not there are symptoms is dependent upon the general state of a man's health at that age. Since there is a trend toward more *diagnosed* prostate cancer in younger and younger men, this leads to the question "What's going on?" From the CDC study that shows the Arizona numbers, it is fairly obvious that there is more to this prostate phenomena than is being publicized.

CDC data exists for most of the other states and relatively speaking, the numbers are the same throughout the U.S. Dr. David Albers, Professor of Medicine, Pharmacology and Public Health at the University of Arizona, noted in comments about the CDC study that "one of the things that people don't understand is that cancer is the Number One killer, *two* times greater than heart disease, for people *under* the age of 65, confirming what we are saying about younger and younger men needing to have PSA screens at their annual physical exams. The sad fact is, however, most men wait until their late 50's or even early 60's before they take serious the advice that regular physical exams need to be a part of every man's life, and now for men, it needs to start at age 40!

TABLE 1

MOST COMMON CANCERS IN MEN (in Arizona)*

*(rates per 100,000 people)

Prostate	114.4
Lungs and bronchus	75.8
Colon and rectum	54.7
Bladder	39.3
Melanomas of the skin	20.1
Non-Hodgkin's lymphoma	19.2
Kidney and renal pelvis	15.0
Mouth and pharynx	12.1
Leukemias	11.3
Pancreas	9.8
Stomach	8.5
Brain and Other Nervous System	7.6
Esophagus	6.9
Liver and Intrahepatic Bile Duct	5.9
Larynx	5.7

*Arizona Republic Newspaper summary of CDC (2002) report, January 12, 2003

NATIONAL STATISTICS

The American Cancer Society (ACS) publishes mortality and morbidity data for all types of cancers and produces the statistics every year for prostate mortality, state by state. For 2003, Table II summarizes the ACS Prostate *Cancer Facts and Figures for 2003:*

TABLE II
Prostate Cancer Statistics

STATE	Estimated New Prostate Cancer Cases Year 2003	Estimated Prostate Cancer Mortality Year 2003	Prostate Cancer Incidence Rates (1995–1999)**	Prostate Cancer Mortality Rates (1995–1999)**
UNITED STATES	220,900	28,900	168.9	33.9
Alabama	4,700	600	93.1	41.9_5
Alaska	200	†	152.2	22.6
Arizona	4,300	600	—	29.9
Arkansas	2,600	300	130.5	37.4
California	$20,500_1$	$2,700_1$	154.3	29.3
Colorado	2,600	300	156.9	30.8
Connecticut	2,800	400	165.6	31.0
Delaware	600	100	172.5_{10}	38.8_9
District of Columbia	600	100	256.6_1	53.7_1
Florida	$15,800_2$	$2,100_2$	—	30.1
Georgia	5,700	700	130.1	41.6_6
Hawaii	900	100	124.1	22.7
Idaho	1,100	100	152.0	35.0
Illinois	$10,100_6$	$1,300_6$	154.2	34.9
Indiana	5,000	700	120.3	35.9
Iowa	2,700	400	152.1	33.1
Kansas	2,100	300	—	31.6
Kentucky	3,300	400	141.5	35.2
Louisiana	3,600	500	170.4	42.1_4
Maine	900	100	147.2	33.4

Maryland	3,900	500	**188.2**[3]	**38.2**[10]
Massachusetts	5,500	700	**174.6**[7]	33.0
Michigan	**7,800**[8]	**1,100**[8]	**183.3**[4]	34.7
Minnesota	4,000	500	**174.0**[8]	35.3
Mississippi	2,900	400	—	**46.0**[2]
Missouri	4,500	600	141.2	32.2
Montana	800	100	164.3	36.0
Nebraska	1,400	200	161.5	29.2
Nevada	1,600	200	99.2	32.8
New Hampshire	900	100	150.2	32.9
New Jersey	**6,600**[10]	**900**[9t]	**188.8**[2]	34.2
New Mexico	1,400	200	147.0	33.4
New York	**14,000**[3]	**1,800**[3]	150.1	32.2
North Carolina	**6,800**[9]	**900**[9t]	146.5	**39.9**[7]
North Dakota	500	100	**179.5**[5]	35.5
Ohio	**9,400**[7]	**1,200**[7]	139.1	34.6
Oklahoma	2,600	300	—	31.2
Oregon	3,200	400	154.8	35.1
Pennsylvania	**12,000**[5]	**1,600**[5]	167.0	34.6
Rhode Island	900	100	172.2	33.9
South Carolina	3,800	500	**177.5**[6]	**43.2**[3]
South Dakota	700	100	—	34.9
Tennessee	4,700	600	106.6	37.1
Texas	**13,200**[4]	**1,700**[4]	148.9	34.3
Utah	1,400	200	**172.8**[9]	37.0
Vermont	300	†	—	36.0
Virginia	5,500	700	145.4	**39.1**[8]

Washington	3,900	500	165.2	30.4
West Virginia	1,700	200	138.0	31.9
Wisconsin	4,500	600	160.3	35.5
Wyoming	400	100	168.0	37.3

Source: American Cancer Society publication *Cancer Facts & Figures 2003.*
*Excludes basal and squamous cell skin cancers and in situ carcinomas except urinary bladder.
†Estimate is 50 or fewer deaths. State death estimates between 51 and 99 were rounded to 100.
**Per 100,000, age adjusted to the 2000 U.S. standard population.
Notes: State estimates may not add to U.S. total due to rounding.
Bold₁ numbers indicate state ranks in national top 10 in given statistic.
t- indicates tie in top 10 statistic.

THE TREND IS YOUNGER ONSET

Dr. Stan Swierzewski, CEO of healthcommunities.com notes that "The younger a man is when he contracts the disease, it seems to be much more aggressive, and if left untreated, will lead to a man's certain demise." (*Today's Arizona Woman,* June 2002). The medical community, at least those physicians who have bothered to think about it, are somewhat baffled by this phenomena and are, therefore, reluctant to publicize information that might be alarming and for which they have few answers. However, it is time that the general public is made aware of the facts, because *prostate cancer rates are increasing at an alarming rate and it is most definitely affecting younger and younger men.*

As discussed before, and to confirm that a trend exists in the current year just as in 2002, according to statistics published by the American Cancer Society in *Surveillance Research* (2001), more than 300,000 men will be diagnosed with prostate cancer. The fact that an increasingly large percentage of those diagnosed will be men *under* the age of 60 has caused urologists and radiation oncologists great concern. Add to this alarming statistic the fact that there has been no known *cause* that has been isolated (i.e. we don't really know how cancer is triggered in the prostate gland), and we have the makings of an epidemic in progress.

The medical community has known for more than a decade that prostate cancer has been consistently increasing in the U.S. During this same period, treatment options for cancers in general, and prostate cancer in particular, have slowly grown as technology has been made available and approved by the American Medical Association and the Federal Drug Administration. Yet the historical treatment techniques used by urologists/surgeons (even for men under the age of 50) is the same as pre-1990; radical prostatectomy (the surgical removal and elimination of the prostate gland) is still the most popular treatment.

It was widely published in 1990 that junk bond financier Michael Milken donated almost $100 million to Cedar Saini hospital in Los Angeles to conduct research on finding out what causes prostate cancer (to start). In 1993, the Milken Foundation formed CaP Cure, the Association for the Cure of Cancer of the Prostate, which has provided more than $100 million to hundreds of clinical trials and research projects aimed at finding a) what causes prostate cancer to start, and b) how to cure prostate cancer. Now, more than a dozen years later, the medical community appears no closer to answering the first question, but one thing that has been shown in answer to question b): *other options for treatment are available that have as good, or statistically better, long-term cure rates as radical prostatectomy* (for men age 40 to 80). The Foundation has also fostered government supported research that has increased from less than $60 million to $430 million in 2002, thus the Foundation has had tremendous impact in the fight on prostate cancer.

And there now is renewed hope that detection methods which predict how aggressive the treatment should be will help doctors determine what treatment should be used when prostate cancer is diagnosed. Researchers at the University of Michigan Medical School announced (*AZ Republic*, October 10, 2002) that they found 55 genes that were more active in metastatic cells than in less-lethal cells with a gene called EZH2, the most active of all.

What they have determined is that the *intensity* of the genes expression, or the prevalence of proteins for which the gene serves as a code, increased as tissue samples progressed from benign to localized to metastatic (i.e. it is when prostate cancer cells have moved outside the prostate capsule and into other parts of the body that it is most dangerous, leading to mortality).

Researchers noted that higher levels of the EZH2 protein were more likely to eventually get the deadlier form of the disease so the gene may be a lethal biomarker which portends aggressiveness. If the EZH2 protein can be monitored in the other PSA (blood) tests used to screen for prostate cancer, it may be a more accurate way of predicting a patient's survival chances than is presently available. That, in turn, leads to more certainty of treatment choice selection which, until now, is like rolling dice.

Judging what treatment option to choose, particularly for younger men, is a major concern, because for younger men the importance of selecting a treatment for their prostate cancer that minimizes side effects cannot be understated. Currently, of all the prostate cancer treatment options available with statistically similar cure rates, the worst side effects accompany radical prostatectomies. Incontinence occurs in almost 50% of men who have the prostate surgically removed, while sexual impotence occurs 90% of the time. While there are experimental procedures such as penial nerve replacements which offer hope for sexual adequacy, there are few incontinence remedies yet available (*Prostate Cancer*, Goodman-1997).

This primer is not the first to reveal what the medical community seems focused on *not* telling you about increasing rates of prostate cancer. Larry Clapp (1997) has written extensively about the foibles of having prostate cancer in a still-available text called *Prostate Health in 90 Days*. Dr. Clapp's text is in its ninth printing (2001) and confirms what Dr. Gordon Grado (Southwest Oncology) and other physicians have seen in their clinical experience: *radical prostatectomy does not always guarantee that cancer will not return.* As this book points out, urologists and general practitioners have not been the first to let the public know why. The problem with Dr. Clapp's book—and one of the reasons more public use has not been made of it—is that it is focused on healing cancer with natural treatment methods. Naturopathic solutions for cancer is just not a topic the AMA and traditional medical community want to endorse, but we have chosen to devote Chapter Five to the subject because we believe that lifestyle does make a difference.

Interestingly, Dr. Clapp's thesis underscores the main limitation to communicating what options exist: the medical community itself. Most General Physicians (GP's) are the first medical doctors to see a prostate problem. This usually occurs because the patient is having urinary symptoms that involve frequent nighttime trips to the bathroom that result in varying degrees of urination difficulty. This is followed by a trip to the GP who administers a digital rectal exam (DRE) which reveals hardening and/or enlargement of the prostate gland. A simple blood test is ordered, with an accompanying Prostate Specific Antigen (PSA) protein readout. If the PSA results are numerically between 0.1 and 2.5, the patient is given medication for infection and asked to return in 30 to 60 days for follow-up. If symptoms persist or if the PSA result is 2.5 or higher, the patient is sent to a urologist for further evaluation.

Or not! Sometimes frequently with men over age 70, urologists and GP's often take a "wait and see" attitude. The patient is told that, in effect, "since cancer is slow-growing, yearly DRE and PSA exams will be the best way to proceed. If the symptoms progress, or worsen, or if the gland continues to grow larger (and/or the PSA results increase numerically in subsequent blood tests), then something might be done. But because prostate glands commonly are enlarged in men over age 50 and since prostate cancer is known to grow so slowly, the chances of having to do anything to treat the cancer are very small." As for the urination problem, a variety of medications are available to help alleviate those symptoms and most urologists are good at prescribing them all! Of course, as noted in the introduction, there is always TURP (treatment).

Just as often, however, for men under the age of 70, the urologist's advice is almost the opposite of "wait and see." This represents an even more serious concern where the incidence of prostate cancer is increasing at the alarming rate it is. This book, therefore, focuses on helping *men of all ages* understand what prostate cancer is and what options there are for treatment. Most importantly for any man, prostate cancer diagnosed early is *not* a death sentence!

And just for inspiration, Southwest Airlines' successful co-founder, chairman, and CEO Herb Kelleher (who was diagnosed in the late 1990's with prostate cancer) appeared at a company dinner recently and swaggered to the podium with a glass of Wild Turkey in one hand and a cigarette in the other. The colorful business leader has a reputation for being truthful, blunt, and at once thought-provoking. When asked about the state of his health and his cancer (and the fact that he was both smoking and drinking alcohol) said,

> "I don't smoke (or drink) with my prostate gland. There may be some men that do that, but I never have!"

It is not the intent of this book to recommend living recklessly, of course. It is, however, important to know what your options are, hopefully to prevent the onset of prostate cancer or, once diagnosed, what to do to live a long and healthy life. It is also not the intent of this book to tell you to *live every day as if it were your last,* as some people advise. In the words of an old high school classmate (Dick Rullman, Class of 1961, Ottumwa, Iowa),

> "I tried living just one day like it was my last, and I worried so much about dying I couldn't enjoy it!"

Read about your options, make the right *informed* choices, and live a long and healthy life!

A recent editorial/opinion in *USA Today* (July 23, 2003) carried the headline: "Prostate Cancer: No Perfect Treatment." It was written by Don Campbell, a *USA Today* publishing company board member who recently had a radical prostate-ctamy and he had this to say:

> "Prostate cancer makes the headlines when celebrity politicians such as Bob Dole and Rudy Giuliani are diagnosed. Macho Joe Sixpack, who doesn't know his prostate from his pituitary, however, often gives those headlines short shrift unless his wife or girlfriend insists he be tested."

Further, in agreement with the premise of this book, Dr Fray Marshall who is chair of the Urology Department at Emory University notes that

> "…men, on the average, are not likely to lobby or be vocal about their prostate, erectile dysfunction, urinary incontinence, loss of manhood and all the implications related to that."

Campbell notes that Hamilton Jordan, former aide to Jimmy Carter, recently chronicled his battle with prostate cancer (plus two other types of cancer) in a best-selling book, *No Such Thing As A Bad Day,* agrees. Jordan said that

> "…women do better than we (men) do at this stuff because they talk about their health and they network more; it's hard to get men to do that."

Throughout this primer we have made it a point to show how little information is publicly available (i.e. that is, information which is highlighted and unavoidable) about prostate cancer, and how important it is for men who have prostate problems *not* to ignore the plethora of options available for decision-making.

THE OSTRICH PRINCIPLE

The popular press is slowly recognizing that men, indeed, are different than women in more than the obvious ways; they don't read as much, and certainly not materials that they aren't already interested in. When they talk over beers at the pub, they avoid medical or sexual topics except as it relates to their prowess, but they especially avoid their own physical conditions. Most men, we realize, practice the "Ostrich Principle," putting their heads in the sand. They would rather not talk about themselves and hope that cancer is something they never have to face. Thus most of them figure that if they don't talk about it they won't get it and they won't have to deal with it.

We need to make general health information available in different ways for men than we do for women. This is even more true for men in their early 40's, who need to include PSA tests in their annual physical exams. This book speaks to that issue, generally, and to men, specifically, about prostate health. Share this with every man you know and we might make a reduction in that 29,000 who will die from prostate cancer next year.

Finally, for additional support for the idea that early screening should begin in men at the age of 35, the Southwest College of Naturopathic Medicine & Health recently made a plea in their winter issue 2003 SCNM Newsletter for men to take care of their prostate health starting at an early age. For men in higher risk categories (i.e. family history, black men), they advise starting PSA screenings at age 25, citing the recent New York postmortem study, which found undiagnosed PC in men in their early twenties.

The medical community seems to be in agreement that PSA testing should begin at an earlier age than has previously been stated publicly. For our purposes here, all the evidence suggests that at least by age 45, every man should have PSA screening, along with a regular physical exam. For high risk men, we suggest starting that at least ten years earlier, by age 35, in order for diagnosis and treatment to be effective while cancer tumors are still contained inside the prostate gland.

And, remember, most men have *no* symptoms, even at ages of 70 or 80, so the PSA screening is today the most likely source of information that will mean the difference between making choices that allow for living a long and healthy life.

1

<u>INTRODUCTION</u>

WHAT THE MEDICAL COMMUNITY KNOWS

The first thing GP's (General Practitioners) usually identify from the DRE (digital rectal exam) in routine physical examinations is BPH (benign prostatic hyperplasia). This is the noncancerous prostate enlargement and/or prostatitis (inflamed prostate) that most men over the age of 50 experience. BPH is usually not a big concern unless it causes the patient to have symptoms (discussed later). What most men hear at the physical exam from the GP is, "Your prostate is enlarged and we will watch it over the next 6 to 12 months. If you have 'symptoms' later, we will do another PSA and go from there." And "By the way, don't worry. It's(usually) benign!" This is where we first hear the term, "watchful waiting" used. And where most men *really* start to worry!

If PSA results are in the high range, the GP may advise the patient to see a urologist for further evaluation. In today's litigious world, no primary care physician likes to take chances with misdiagnosing a problem that might be as serious as prostate cancer. Because urologists conduct digital rectal exams (DRE) frequently, they tend to have a much better "feel" for prostates (pun intended), and their diagnosis of what problem the patient may have is usually much more accurate than the General Practitioner (GP). Still, the urologist will usually request that more than one PSA (blood test result) be taken before identifying and diagnosing the problem completely.

The PSA—or prostate specific antigen—is a measure in nanograms per milliliter of the blood content of a protein known to be produced by the prostate gland, *sort of* in response to cancer cells being formed or proliferating…*sort of.*

Historically, if PSA results are lower than 4.0 (nanograms per milliliter), most urologists (and GP's) will have a "wait and see" attitude, although they may want another PSA in cases where the PSA result is between 2.5 and 4.0, just to see if it's stable or if it is rising. But remember, PSA levels only estimate how *likely* a man is to have prostate cancer, although it does not always *predict* that cancer is present. Different doctors might approach the diagnostics differently; it's why we recommend getting more than one opinion when borderline PSA results are consistent over time.

A recent study published in the *Journal of the American Medicine Association* (JAMA) in July, 2003 found that men, particularly men under age 50, who had PSA results of less than 2.9 were still at risk. The results indicated that *not screening men with PSA's between 2.4 and 2.9 resulted in missing cancer in as many as 60%* of those who were retested. This is particularly alarming when you consider that biopsies are usually not recommended unless PSA's are greater than (about) 4.0 in most men.

An editorial in the same *JAMA* issue recommends "wait and watch" for those men, somewhat contradicting the authors of the study, all of which leads to further confusion for the man whose PSA is in that "gray" range 2.5 to 3.9. Thus it is no wonder that men don't pursue second and third opinions when their diagnosis is positive!

Some studies have shown that as many as 25% of men with prostate cancer have a low PSA (NCCN, 2001). In one case, known personally to the authors of this book, a 44 year old man in Phoenix, Arizona had increasingly severe symptoms of nighttime urination problems over 6 to 8 months before going for a DRE and PSA evaluation. Two GP's and two urologists said he had *early* BPH and evaluated consistently low PSA results (i.e. less than 0.8!) to mean "wait and watch" with "not even the slight possibility of cancer being present," as stated by one doctor. Subsequent evaluation at Cedars Siani Hospital revealed almost total tumor in the young man's prostate and immediate surgery was recommended (Cedars, 2001).

Interestingly, a recent study undertaken at the Oregon Health and Science University Cancer Institute demonstrates the confused state of information and "mixed-messages" that are provided about prostate cancer to the general public. In a study that looked at more than 1,200 men with PSA levels ranging from 4 to 10 who had biopsies between 1993 and 2000, the Director of Urologic Oncology at the Portland Veterans' Affairs Medical Center, Dr. Mark Garzotto, discussed the findings in the popular press.

After a man has the PSA result that the urologist or GP says is in the high range (i.e. above 2.5), but not statistically different than previous PSA results (taken over several months time), the doctor is likely to conclude that "just watching it" (i.e. watchful waiting) for a few months is the best course of action. Medication might be prescribed for the urinary symptoms, or in the case of a patient that had no urinary symptoms but whose PSA was in the high range in a routine physical exam, the doctor might request another PSA in 30 to 60 days. Or as in the case where the PSA appears to be climbing slowly over three or four month's PSA tests, the option of doing a biopsy on the prostate might be discussed.

Good urologists will not "prescribe" a biopsy, but rather *suggest* to the patient that it is his choice; a biopsy, they will be advised, however, will be definitive almost 100% of the time…*"almost…"*

The choice is clearly left to the patient whether or not to actually have a biopsy done, because biopsies (unbeknown to the patient) carry a risk that the urologist does not want to be liable for, that of spreading cancer cells that are otherwise "contained" in the prostate. More about this later.

As discussed before, a urologist also may say that because prostate cancer is *"slow growing,"* there is plenty of time to decide whether a biopsy is warranted or not. Unfortunately, that conclusion—while being statistically accurate—is based on the history of prostate cancer growth in men *over* 70 where life expectancy is short (i.e. average lifetime is 76 years) and men usually die from some other cause (Schachter, World Health OnLine, 2002) For younger men who face the possibility of cancer, getting a biopsy sooner rather than later may be crucial to treatment while the cancer cells are still contained in the prostate gland (and have not migrated to other parts of the body).

CANCER INDICATORS, PSA, BIOPSIES AND GLEASON SCORES

According to Bostwick Laboratories (www.bostwicklaboratories.com), the Gleason grading system is as important as PSA in understanding tumor stages. The Gleason score is a sum of the two most prevalent patterns detected by the pathologist, ranging from 2 (least aggressive) to 10 (most aggressive). Commonly, the TNN system is used to "grade" tumors, with 'T' representing the size of the primary tumor, 'N' representing the involvement of lymph nodes, and 'M' being metastisis (migration) outside the gland. Both these Gleason measures are important in understanding prostate cancer (tumors) and the Bostwick Laboratories web site offers a most excellent explanation that every diagnosed man needs to know.

The procedure for conducting a biopsy of the prostate gland incorporates the use of hollow needles inserted into the prostate which extract tissue samples, usually 6 to 8 in number, which are sent to a laboratory where they are evaluated for cancer cells. This almost painless procedure is usually conducted in the urologist's office using a computer probe inserted up the rectal canal to map the prostate. The urologist then utilizes the computer image in snaking the needle device up the rectal canal where s/he inserts and removes the needles to extract tissue for laboratory evaluation. "Extract" is the operative word; the procedure actually tears or rips the tiny tissue culture from the gland as it is withdrawn. Because the urethra winds its way right through the prostate gland, bleeding insues that manifests itself in the urine for several hours, and sometimes days afterwards. This is, however, normal and should clear up in a day or two at most.

What is important to know about this procedure, however, is that the needle insertion/retraction pathway is left from inside the prostate to the outside of the gland, whereby any cancer cells might be able to migrate and make their way into other parts of the body. This is the "biopsy risk" that urologists do not like to discuss that was mentioned before. At this time, there are no good alternatives to this procedure for definitively learning if cancer is present in the prostate gland. Best advice, therefore, is to ask a lot of questions, talk to more than one urologist, and chose the most experienced practicioner that gives you straight answers to your questions.

AFTER THE BIOPSY: If the results are positive

Urologists who do the needle biopsies know the probability of cancer cells migrating through this procedure is low, but they prefer that patients not know about it at all. When biopsy results confirm that cancer cells are present, a radical prostatectomy (i.e. surgical procedure to remove the prostate gland) is frequently recommended, and there is usually little discussion about the probability that the cancer might metasticize at a later time. In fact, most doctors tell patients that surgically removing the prostate gland is the *only* sure way to eliminate the cancer. Thus patients who choose to have a radical prostatectomy and then find some years later that their cancer has metastacized (returned) elsewhere in their body may never know that the biopsy they had years before was possibly the way their cancer spread. This would be the "horse was already out of the barn" corollary urologists/surgeons use for why cancer reappeared after the prostate gland was removed!

It is for this reason that patients should not wait too long after a biopsy to decide on what treatment should be done. This is true no matter what treatment option, including non-surgical procedures, is chosen, since the migration pathways are open from the needle biopsy procedure the moment the biopsies are taken.

Patients choosing to seek other medical opinions about treatment options generally find out from oncology radiologists who specialize in prostate cancer treatment that the risk of the biopsy pathway needs to be followed quickly by external beam radiation treatment(s) so the migration is stemmed before it reaches the outside layers of the gland. Even for men who choose surgery, or radical prostatectomy, external beam radiation might be recommended to kill cancer cells outside, but in the general area of the prostate gland, before surgery is performed. The urologist/surgeon is oftentimes reluctant to make such a recommendation, fearing opening up liability issues that might be difficult to defend if cancer later returns after treatment—years later. (See also a later discussion about a 2003 Mayo Clinic study that deals with this topic)

Just as often, men being the reluctant animal they are to discuss anything as personal as medical problems with their "sexual system," would rather trust the advice of the urologist and not seek second or third opinions about treatment options. That is why about 60% to 80% of the time, surgery is recommended and no other opinions are sought by the patient. Men just want to get the "problem" fixed and get on with their lives with no "personal" discussions to embarrass them.

It is the opinion of the authors of this book that proper communication with the general population about the increasingly large numbers of prostate cancers diagnosed and the misinformation (or intentional lack of it) being given out by the medical community warrants a critical look. It is to this end that the authors of this book have compiled the resources and data that are intended to enlighten men who are concerned about their prostate health.

AFTER THE BIOPSY: When Results Are Negative

It is just as important to know what it means to get a "negative" biopsy result. Generally, a low PSA result (i.e. a numerical result less than 3.0) will not be considered a potential problem and the examining physician may recommend that no biopsy be performed. "Just watch it for six months and do another PSA with DRE…" is a typical recommendation. However, if the patient is having classic symptoms of frequent night-time trips to the bathroom and the prostate is enlarged and/or feels "hard" to the touch in the DRE, a biopsy may be recommended when PSA would not otherwise indicate that a potential problem exists.

Whenever a biopsy procedure is done, the cautionary information provided previously should be heeded; if cancer cells are present (even microscopic-sized cells), there is an increased risk that they may be provided a pathway outside the gland via the needle paths in the biopsy. Where those cells might not have been a problem inside the gland for years (or perhaps never), once allowed to migrate outside to other parts of the body, microscopic cancer cells represent a greater risk of full-blown carcinogenicity in other parts of the body.

There are cases also where men had PSA results on subsequent examinations of less than 1.0, but the symptoms (enlarged gland, hard surfaces, frequent bathroom urination trips; etc.) were so overwhelming that a biopsy revealed that cancer in the prostate was present. Thus a "normal" PSA does not always mean that results are "negative," and the doctor should consult with men who find themselves in this situation to determine what steps should be taken. It is frequently the case that the urologist recommends a "wait and see" period before repeating the tests (including biopsies that have been negative). A man finding himself in this situation should seek second and third opinions from other urologists and radiologists who specialize in prostate treatment.

NEGATIVE BIOPSY RESULTS: Does It Mean Cancer Is *NOT* Present?

There are also many documented cases of men having all the symptoms who go in for a biopsy only to reveal that no cancer cells were present. Even when PSA results are sometimes ten, twenty or higher, when the biopsy results did not find cancer cells present, what normally is advised by the physicians is "wait and watch," then have a PSA again in six months or a year. Unfortunately, in case after case when the patient returns with the same (or statistically similar) PSA result in six months, another biopsy is recommended.

There are men who have had this occur over a three to five year period and had a biopsy each subsequent time, only to receive negative results. But the prostate gland, after having more than a dozen or two needle biopsies, is scarred and even a higher risk of transporting microscopic cancer cells outside the gland with *no diagnostic method of learning if that is happening or not.* In most of the cases reviewed for this book where this situation has occurred, ultimate MRI and PET scans showed the presence of tumor(s) in the prostate gland, even where the biopsy results were still considered to be negative.

SUMMARY

Most men are reluctant to go to doctors with problems that they are having in those "unmentionable" places on their bodies. When it comes to the prostate gland, men are even less inclined to seek medical help, fearing the embarrassment of their perceived "situation" will be humiliating. Thus problems with frequent and incomplete night time urination, discomfort in the penis or rectal areas, or sexual dysfunction are likely to be ignored until there seems to be no other way to get relief. By then, men who find out they have an enlarged prostate gland and an abnormally high PSA just want to get a "fix" to the problem and live a normal life again. The options for prostate cancer sufferers, however, are more than just radical prostatectomy, and getting second and third medical opinions is a key to making the right therapy choice.

2

In this chapter you will learn about…

Diagnosis and Prognosis:

What the Studies Show: You Need to Know!

Most Common Treatment Options Today

What Surgery and Prostate Gland Removal Mean

What External Beam Radiation Can and Cannot do

What Brachytherapy (Radioactive Seed Implants) Can and Cannot Do

Cancer Indicators, PSA, Biopsies and Gleason Scores

Popular Therapies

Hormonal Therapy

INTRODUCTION

Numerous urologists who do needle placements (only) for radiologists who insert radiation seeds in the treatment known as brachytherapy will tell you that they don't keep statistics on the patients. They will tell you that "it's the Radiologist/Oncologist who wants to know…" the success rate. When you inquire at hospitals where radical prostatectomies are performed, you will find that the statistics are not available (except to need-to-know doctors), and this is just an extension of the problem discussed before: communicating to the patient; the community is pretty much restricted to whatever doctors want (or the AMA).

For this book, therefore, we used studies and literature that was taken from public domain sites on the internet, clinics that do prostate cancer research and treatment, and the very large (and well documented) data base of Southwest Oncology, which consists of more than 7000 prostate cancer patients. Thus what you read about here is real-world, timely, up-to-date (at the end of 2003, unless noted in the text), and is intentionally written at the lay-public level with as few medical jargon terms as possible.

It is anticipated, also, that our biggest critics will be from the medical community. We encourage debate and, most of all for men of all ages, the medical community needs to be more forthcoming on this increasingly controversial problem. If we succeed in providing options to even a handful of men, we will have fulfilled our goal.

DIAGNOSIS AND PROGNOSIS: What the Studies Show

When we looked back at the thousands of brachytherapy patients treated by Dr. Grado and Dr. Ragde over the past fifteen years, we noticed that the patients, on the average. were getting younger. Prostate cancer has, however, historically been called "the disease for old men"; if a man lives long enough—say into his 90's—there is a greater than 90% probability that he will have cancer of the prostate. But it was also thought that such cancers didn't usually appear until men were well into their 60's or mid-70's. Even then, because prostate cancer has been seen as very slow growing, there was always the option to wait and watch, perhaps treating the (slow urination) symptoms while patients eventually succumbed of some other malady. Life spans for men, after all, is still mid-70's, so taking a slow and deliberate approach to prostate cancer seemed the right approach in a majority of cases.

In the last decade of the 20th century, however, the average age of prostate cancer patients declined (Southwest Oncology, 2001). In a study quoted by Dr. Schachter (Health World OnLine, 2001), careful pathological examinations of the prostate glands during the autopsies of men killed in accidents revealed some alarming figures. According to Schachter, "the study showed that the incidence of microscopic prostate cancer was 80% in men between the ages 70 and 80 years old, 40% in men between 50 and 60 years old, 34% in men between 40 and 50 years old, and 27% in men between 30 and 40 years old." These are alarming numbers, even realizing that they refer to *microscopic* prostate cancer and not to *clinical* prostate cancer (which is diagnosed when a person is alive).

The Southwest College of Naturopathic Medicine, SCNM Newsletter (www.scnm.edu, Winter-2003 issue) also reported that a recent New York post-mortem study found undiagnosed prostate cancer in men in their early twenties, so the medical community at least realizes this is no longer just a disease that older men get. With new diagnostics technology arriving every day, we are coming to realize that PC is a bigger risk to men than anyone ever thought possible.

The autopsies used in the studies quoted were conducted for other reasons than to compile prostate information so the conclusions drawn about cancer cells in the prostates of younger men are certainly unbiased, But they are startling and illuminating. What this says for the researchers who are trying to find out what causes the spontaneous emission of cancer cell growth in the prostate is *such microscopic cancer cells may be present in a large segment of the male population,* and isolating the trigger mechanism for onset is more crucial than thought, particularly if we are ever to eliminate or eradicate prostate cancer.

The idea that prostate cancer screening should begin in men at the age of 50 is supported by, among others, the American Cancer Society, NCCN, and the American Urological Association (UAU), and should occur annually because early detection of prostate cancer can lead to successful treatment. A recent federally funded study concluded that "the risk of prostate cancer is so low for these men that checking once every two years, or even every five years, is enough to find cancer in time." (__AP; May 21, 2002)

The study results were reviewed by one of its authors, University of Colorado professor E. D. Crawford, at the Orlando American Society of Clinical Oncology on May 20, 2002 where he noted that the recommendations for further testing should be based on PSA levels. He said the study concludes that where PSA readings are between zero and 1.0, a man can wait 5 years to have another test. If reading is between 1 and 2.0, he can wait two years to have another test, and those whose readings are between 2 and 4.0 should continue to have annual tests. "If (the study guidelines are) followed," Dr. E. D. Crawford noted, "(this) will mean much less testing for the majority of men…"

It should be noted, however, that all of this, (*not* overtly highlighted in the study) was an attempt to reduce the *cost* of screening for prostate cancer, as noted in the fine print which said that if the guidelines are followed, the number of PSA tests per year would be cut in half, and a savings (to insurance companies?) of $500 Million to $1 Billion would be realized nationwide.

This study and its conclusions are obviously at odds with the statistics on the incidence of prostate cancer. It may be an artifact of how the study was set up, or it may be "creative statistics" being used to show a way to reduce medical costs. It was a "federally funded" study, but little information is available on what agency sponsored it or for what reason the study was conducted. Common sense (and a look at "creative statistics") would show, however, that reducing the number of PSA tests performed only reduces the number of "potential" cancers detected. If you don't look for it, you won't find it, so avoiding the $10-$20 PSA lab cost in yearly physical exams (i.e. saving the insurance companies $50 to $100 over five annual exams) is likely to result in a much higher incidence of positive results in men 55 years of age. The percentage of those diagnosed men having "confined" prostate cancer at that point in their lives will likely be less than if it had been screened (and detected) five years earlier. Is it worth it? Ask the man who follows this guideline *after* he finds out his prostate cancer is unconfined what *he* thinks of his doctor's (and this study's) advice.

As a result of the data compiled for this book, the authors believe PSA screens should begin *even earlier* than is currently recommended. Rather than age 50, as has been recommended by the ACS and other medical and oncology organizations, we believe the proper time to include PSA is between the ages of 40 and 45. If there is a family history of prostate cancer, age 40 would be recommended, and where PSA results at that time were less than 1.0, screening every other year until age 50 would be the recommendation. Of course if symptoms manifest themselves during the ages 40 to 50, more diagnostics are required. After age 50, the data suggests that *all* men should have an annual physical examination with *both* a DRE and PSA. Nothing in studies or the literature utilized in the research for this book changes that recommendation.

Again, it's communication that is important. As noted before, most middle-aged men haven't even thought about prostate health at the age of 40. And yes, 40 is middle-aged, like it or not! But making it through the "second half" of your life requires understanding what options are available (for such threats to your health as cancer). Therefore, making the information available and publicizing it to men early is just as important as publicizing breast cancer information to women at an early stage. We believe that men have the intelligence to take care of their own health by age 40 and that prostate cancer information is just as important to communicate to them as are the so called "fitness" and "workout" commercials aimed at the aging "boomers" every day in the media. Let's be sure we are communicating the *right* message; "Fit at 40 and beyond" should be our mantra. Prostate health should be a part of that mantra, also.

OTHER TREATMENTS AND STUDIES OF INTEREST

At this writing, a very promising vaccine is being developed by clinical researchers at Johns Hopkins. The FDA says it is "promising" and expects to approve it within a couple of years. Potentially, what a vaccine would mean would be that like other childhood diseases which vaccines have eradicated, the vaccine could be administered at a young (yet-to-be-determined) age, and like polio, the world (i.e. *all* men!) could quit worrying about it. Unfortunately, the optimistic speculation may not live up to the expectations, so in the meantime we must keep trying to find the cause while spreading the word about the variety of successful treatments available—for the foreseeable future.

Also, as noted earlier in this chapter, in another study conducted at the University of Michigan Medical School in 2001/2002, researchers examined tumor cells taken from prostate cancer patients. They found 55 genes that were more active in metastatic cells than in less-lethal cells. A gene called EZH2 showed that its activity increased as the disease progressed, and patients who showed higher levels of the EZH2 protein were more likely to get the deadlier form of the disease.

Dr. A.M. Chinnaiyan, an assistant professor of pathology and a lead investigator in the study noted that

> "…it suggests that this is a lethal biomarker, that portends aggressiveness…and, if a test can be developed, EZH2 protein levels could be used to decide which patients need aggressive treatment, including radiation and/or surgery."

The study, published in the October 11, 2002 edition of *Nature*, also points out that many men over 60 years of age are receiving unnecessary surgery and other treatments for prostate cancer that is unlikely to spread…and that this new biomarker may be one answer for screening out those men who should have further treatment from those who should not. At this early date, however, the EZH2 screening tool may be unavailable in most hospitals, so it remains to be seen where this research will lead.

COMMON TREATMENT OPTIONS TODAY:
The Radical Prostatectomy (Surgery)

As mentioned before, the most common treatment being recommended today for prostate cancer is radical prostatectomy (i.e. surgical removal of the prostate gland). Remember,: it's not called "radical" for nothing. For men who are older than 75 or 80, this may be a good option if certain conditions exist—assuming, once again, that the cancer is found to be confined to the prostate gland and enlargement of the gland is not correctable any other way.

Condition #1: Sex is no longer important or necessary in your life.

It's generally thought that men in their twilight years have little or no sex life. From studies and reports based on retirement communities in the southwestern U.S. (i.e. remember the sexy Sun City, Arizona residents caught having "relations" outdoors in 2000?) this may be a false assumption. GP's and urologists know that healthy men over the age of 70 are likely to still be having sex at least once or twice a month, sometimes more frequently. Men between the ages of 50 and 70 are likely to have sex even more frequently, so for a man of *any* age (not just 75 or older) who is diagnosed with prostate cancer and a radical prostatectomy is recommended, answering this question should be the first priority.

Condition #2: Impotence will be almost certain, but so will incontinence.

After a Radical Prostatectomy, incontinence occurs in 90% of all men for a period lasting from three months to forever. The severity of incontinence may range from total loss of control to partial loss of control (at each urination event), but 40% to 50% of all men who have a radical prostatectomy have incontinence *forever*. Yes, they do have diapers now for adults, but is that what you really want to have happen? Think about it!

Condition #3: Radical Prostatectomy does not guarantee that cancer won't return later:

(…even though most urologists will say it is the only sure "treatment" that eliminates cancer)

For many reasons, removal of the prostate gland does not guarantee that cancer cells have not already migrated outside the prostate gland (i.e. it is unconfined) before surgery. One of the ways this happens, as discussed earlier, is during the biopsy, but there are other reasons, and most of them will never be discussed with the patient.

When a radical prostatectomy is performed, the layers of the gland are peeled away like the layers of an onion until only the outer "skin" is left attached to the various tissue that once held the gland in place. If cancer cells are present in this layer of skin, they are immediately available to migrate to other parts of the body. thus, removal of the gland can still leave behind cancer cells that will grow to live another day in another place in the body. In fact, they may be in the groin area within days of the biopsy being performed, but certainly they can be "spread" in the surgical process of radical prostatectomy. Even the surgeons will not discount that possibility, preferring instead to point to the "10 year survival" rates of 80+% of their patients. The question is, when you are under the age of 45 to 50, is ten years enough?

TWO PROCEDURES ARE COMMON

According to doctors at the Mayo Clinic, two procedures are available for a prostatectomy: retropubic and perineal surgery. In retropubic surgery, the gland is taken out through an incision in the lower abdomen that typically runs from just below the navel to about an inch above the penis. It's the most common form of prostate removal, because lymph nodes surrounding the prostate can be removed and tested to make sure the cancer hasn't spread. Plus, the procedure gives the surgeon better access to the prostate, making it easier to save the nerve bundles that control erection, although they may not always be undamaged.

Perineal surgery utilizes an incision made between the anus and the scrotal sac, which holds the testicles. This method generally involves less bleeding, and heavier men recover sooner, but because the approach is much more difficult than retropubic surgery, it is much more difficult to locate and save the nerve bundles. Of course lymph nodes are not accessible in this method, and that is the reason this procedure is less commonly used.

Newer robotic procedures are being used now which allow the procedure to be done with less pain, less loss of blood and no scars. According to doctors at Scottsdale (Arizona) Shea Healthcare hospital (*AZ Republic Supplement*, 6/2/03), the daVinci Surgical System provides three-dimensional magnification not available with traditional laparoscopic equipment and utilizes 3 computerized robotic arms—one with a 3-D camera and the other two with precision surgical instruments. The pencil-sized arms are placed inside the patient through small incisions and are maneuvered by the surgeon who sits at a console a few feet from the operating table. This robotic procedure causes less discomfort and a return to normal activity more rapidly than a traditional laparoscopic prostatectomy procedure. More information on the promising daVinci surgical procedure is in Chapter 6.

It is important to note, however, that success rates in preserving continence and erectile function appear to be similar between prostatectomies done with the daVinci method and those done through open surgery, although recent papers in the *Journal of Urology* (Nov. '02) indicate in prospective studies that Robotic RP patients rarely have incontinence or erectile disfunction longer than two years after surgery. So while expectations for better outcomes may or may not be increased with the daVinci surgical procedures, the discomforts of the surgical process itself are much reduced.

It should be also noted that not every urologist/surgeon is trained on robotic systems, so the availability of this procedure should cause the interested patient to seek out more than one opinion on what surgery (if any) is right for them. The answers you get, in part, may depend upon the experience of the surgeon you talk to, so seek out more than one opinion!

For the man who understands the three conditions, it should be easier to make a decision to go ahead with a radical prostatectomy (or *not*), but for most men, this should be a *last* choice. That is the reason we recommend getting second and third opinions before making a life-changing decision.

Even for the man who appears to have cancer cells outside the prostate gland, the choice for radical prostatectomy is still not definite. In fact, for the man in this situation, such surgery might be totally unnecessary, and working on finding and eliminating the cancer cells that have migrated outside the gland should be a first priority. (This is what is intended when surgeons administer hormone shots, or hormonal therapy, discussed later, in Chapter Six). Again, there are different options for the man in this circumstance, and obtaining second and third opinions is absolutely essential.

Remember also that even recognized treatment centers like the Mayo Clinic understand that radical prostatectomy patients have a nearly 30% reoccurrence rate (www.mayoclinic.com; 2001). Again, this kinds of statistics should send up red flags; explore all your options before deciding on prostate cancer (treatment) solutions.

OTHER OPTIONS: External Beam Radiation and Brachytherapy

In a later chapter, there is a discussion of cutting edge therapies now under development in Europe and the US. Those therapies may be an option for men, even today, under certain circumstances. However, the *proven* therapies (i.e. those that are showing cure results of 80% to 97% in men treated since the early '90's) are called

External Beam Radiation

Brachytherapy (Radioactive Seed Implants)

Radical Prostatectomy

These three treatments for prostate cancer are statistically about equal in their success at stopping cancer (for ten years). That is, all three of these treatments have been tracked in various studies and have been found to be about equally effective for men living ten years afterwards (or for men who died during that time of some other cause). In other words, for all practical purposes choosing one or the other of the three treatments had the same results: cancer was "cured" (i.e. "cured" means the patients lived ten more years after treatment).

The difference in treatment choice, therefore, was in the quality of life that each therapy left the patient with after treatment. As explained in the discussion on Radical Prostatectomy earlier, side effects of that treatment are a *major* consideration.

If E-Beam treatments are conducted over several weeks, as is typically recommended (i.e. 5 to 7 weeks, E-Beam radiation 5 days out of seven each week), there is usually "burning" of sensitive tissues near and surrounding the prostate gland that last several months.* In this procedure, radiation is delivered by a beam from a large machine placed over the body. Unfortunately, these "external beams" do more than destroy cancerous cells; they can damage healthy tissue in the same area, and that is why the first step in radiation therapy is to map out the areas in your body to receive radiation.

Three-dimensional scans show the location of the prostate and surrounding organs, then computer imaging software allows a radiation therapist to rotate the picture in any direction to find the best angles to direct the beams. For External Beam Radiation, also called "E-Beam," side effects are related to the amount and number of E-Beam treatments the patient undergoes. In addition, side effects also may be related to the location of the tumor(s) in the prostate gland and the pathway the E-Beam travels to reach the tumor(s).

In some cases, for example, where tumor(s) are near the inside surface of the gland and in close proximity to the anus, the E-Beam actually "radiates" or burns areas around the sensitive anus tissue as it irradiates the cancer cells inside the prostate gland. This patient will suffer pain and discomfort in the groin and anus area for weeks, or even months afterwards. Doctors recommending this treatment are beginning to explore different treatment schemes now in an effort to minimize this after-effect, but the man choosing this therapy should expect several weeks or even months of after-effects.

It is also true that oncology/radiologists are using E-Beam treatments before Brachytherapy just to ensure that cancer cells that might have migrated outside the prostate gland (but remain in the general vacinity) are destroyed before radiation "seeds" are implanted. This might involve only 2 or 3 E-Beam treatments of a minute each that will usually not result in side effects that full E-Beam treatment promote, although tumors located at or near the prostate surface might cause E-Beam burning to the soft tissues, as noted before.

The Mayo Clinic (www.mayoclinic.com) notes that sexual impotence occurs in 30% to 50% of men treated with external beam radiation, although that is not substantiated in other studies. Incontinence, however, is rare in E-Beam patients.

> (***Note:** One patient interviewed for this text had only two E-Beam treatments, instead of the normal 4–6 weeks, just prior to getting the radioactive seed implants, and a year later had bleeding from radiation "burns" on the inside of the colon where the E-Beam passed through tissue surrounding the prostate.
>
> A second patient interviewed nearly 2 years after undergoing 5 weeks of E-Beam treatments, followed by brachytherapy, continued to experience severe pain and bleeding in the colon and rectum accompanied by intermittent incontinence and some sexual dysfunction.)

BRACHYTHERAPY

The other type of radiation therapy that has become more and more popular is brachytherapy. In this treatment, ultrasound-guided needles are used to inject rice-sized radioactive "seeds" into the prostate around the tumors. These "seeds"—either made up of iodine 150, palladium, or strontium—contain just enough radiation (i.e. about twice the dose of the E Beam) that the tumors are bombarded (for months after treatment), but healthy surrounding tissues are not affected.

The procedure is conducted in an operating room on an out-patient basis and takes about 90 minutes. Just as with surgery, the patient is anesthesized and needles containing the "seeds" are inserted through the parineam and into the prostate around the tumor(s) that were identified previously in an ultrasound exam. In the recovery room after the implants are finished, the catheter is removed and the patient goes home, sometimes resuming a regular schedule the next day after treatment.

Because the procedure for inserting the radioactive seeds into the prostate gland is similar to the biopsy procedure, scar tissue will be gradually formed around the insertion pathways inside the gland. For the immediate 48 hours following the brachytherapy procedure, the urination of blood and a stinging sensation occurs throughout the length of the penis with each urination event. The blood in the urine eventually subsides, although it may persist for as much as a week or two, but the stinging sensation ebbs and flows throughout the penis and into the bladder for weeks or months after the procedure. (Of all the after-effects, patients interviewed for this research said this "burning" sensation and its variations were the most annoying).

Because the prostate gland provides the "pump" and seminal fluid for ejaculation of the sperm in male orgasim, the first few times after treatment that a man has sex, the fluid will be bloody. Again, as with urination, this blood content diminishes over the first few weeks after treatment until no trace is seen. In most men, even though there is a fairly great amount of blood in the seminal ejaculation the first few times, there is very little pain and sex *should* be resumed almost without concern in a very short time span after the implant procedure.(*)

> *(Note: The authors of this primer queried Dr. Grado about how soon sex should be resumed after brachytherapy surgery and he replied, "We prefer that patients wait until after they have been discharged from the hospital!")

The emphasis on "should" be resumed is intentional; in order to ensure that the prostate gland still functions properly, it is recommended that frequent sex is preferable to infrequent. Ejaculation helps keep the prostate gland functioning while the scar tissue is building, and it is thought that it will function better and longer into the future, if sex and ejaculation are resumed soon after treatment.

As noted before, one thing that all men who have had brachytherapy experience is the continued "burning" sensation throughout the entire length of the penis whenever urinating. This is a "sensation" that can only be understood by men who have experienced it, but suffice it to say, it manifests itself in the head of the penis sometimes and sometimes throughout the length of the penis (feeling like it goes all the way back up into the bladder!). The sensation, usually very strong in the first days and weeks after treatment, varies in intensity over time and lasts (in some men) a year or more.

The "flow" of urine also varies in the brachytherapy patient. In the early weeks after treatment, flow will be difficult sometimes, especially at night after sleep has induced a relaxed state to the bladder and urethra. Prescription medication can relieve these symptoms but will still be required in most men for months following the procedure.

One thing is for certain, while these side effects are sometimes painful and generally annoying, they do diminish over time. Thus use of brachytherapy as a treatment of choice to eliminate cancer cells in the prostate gland should be considered to have the *least* side effects of concern (of the three most common treatments reviewed in this text) for long term health and quality of life.

Dr. David Beyer, an MD/Brachytherapist who pioneered seed implantation in the late 1980's at Scottsdale (Arizona) Healthcare, noted in a recent supplement to the *Arizona Republic* (6/2/03), that "…brachytherapy has several advantages to surgery or external radiation, (such as)

* Fewer side effects than other treatments

* Is less invasive than major surgery

* Is less damaging to surrounding tissue

* Has been proven effective against cancer (in the Prostate Gland)

Dr. Beyer notes that

"…we have long term follow-up data (now)" and "the chance of patients being cured are as good as with any other treatment method."

HORMONAL THERAPY

A discussion of treatment therapies would be incomplete without discussing Hormonal (Depravation) Therapy, which is most certainly a well-established form of treatment for various and specific stages of prostate cancer. According to the Prostate Institute of America web site (July, 2003), the historical treatment of choice was to conduct a bilateral orchietctomy (removal of the testicles) to reduce or eliminate the male hormone called "androgen" production which is responsible for tumor growth.

This may seem a radical step to take, but for some patients whose cancer has spread outside the prostate capsule, it is/was a lifesaver. Recently, combination androgen ablation therapy was introduced and commercially available to maximize androgen blockade. Here's how this type of therapy works: there are two major organs in the human body that excrete male hormone. The major source is testicles, and the second source is the adrenal glands. Types of drugs specifically for blocking the hormones excreted by the testicles are called LHRH agonists, such as Lupron or Zoladex. Flutamide or Casodex are the primary drugs used for adrenal gland hormone blockades.

There are some known complications on these drugs. Some experience hot flashes, diarrhea, insomnia, liver function damage and untold effects on the cardiovascular system and some men experience noticeable enlargement of the breast areas. But for men in these circumstances, there are few treatment choices and strict supervision of hormonal deprivation therapy by a specialized physician is vital.

The Prostate Institute of America notes that combination androgen ablation therapy can be used as a primary form of treatment if someone has advanced cancer and it most likely will work, but effective treatment results show no cancer growth for 3 to 5 years, then usually tumor growth starts again. Thus it is important to know the pros and cons before choosing this treatment and understand how progress should be carefully monitored.

The Institute also notes on its website that "the major problem of prostate cancer treatment is under-estimation of the disease, or thinking it's understaged." In studies cited, they note that on the basis of their radical surgery (prostatectomy) experiences, approximately 50% of all cancers thought to be localized in the prostate have actually escaped out of the prostate capsule. (Note: they do not say or suggest when cancer cells might have migrated outside the capsule; see Chapter One discussion of biopsy and brachytherapy cell migration.)

The Institute notes that

> "…since androgen blockade therapy can decrease the size of the tumor and the size of the prostate itself, the chances of an unexpected tumor extension outside of prostate at the time of surgery is minimized (downstaged)."

It is unclear if the Institute made this observation to further enhance the desirability of seeking a prostatectomy as the treatment of choice or if the observation was for information purposes.

Whatever the reasons, selection of hormonal therapy (with or without combining it with another treatment) should be considered only in cases where the tumors are thought to have spread outside the prostate capsule. For this reason, most statistics on this type of therapy have come from men over the age of their late 70's and may have to be reevaluated for men in their younger 50's to early 70's.

SUMMARY

Being diagnosed with a prostate problem means that a journey into uncharted medical territory is about to be undertaken. What direction is chosen is individual circumstance-driven; each man needs to begin the journey with the goal of living a healthy life, no matter what the diagnosis shows. In order to take the right steps toward that goal, information needs to be obtained and opinions of medical professionals sought that will lead to a successful outcome. If cancer is diagnosed in this journey, treatment options are available which can have a high probability of meeting the goal expectations.

A recent article in the AARP magazine, *My Generation* (July-August 2002) highlights the journey taken by author/writer Hal Ackerman when he learned during a routine physical that he had prostate cancer. It is one man's view, very well-written and clearly descriptive, of the ebb and flow of emotions a man feels as he goes through the process of dealing with prostate cancer. Ackerman's ability to paint his emotions in graphic color that can easily be understood are outstanding and we recommend the article to anyone with an interest in prostate cancer. His description of getting the biopsy results, while not necessarily accurate, deals head-on with the feelings those dreaded words evoke:

> "'...you've got cancer...!'"

These are the words no one ever expects to hear, and thus how one deals with those results becomes the foundation for making treatment choices based on many, many opinions by the medical community. It is highly recommended reading! For example, Ackerman retained his sense of humor, even though there are serious issues to debate.

On Radical Prostatectomy (surgical removal of the prostate gland), Ackerman quipped,

> "...given the proximity of the prostate to the male anatomy, you're cutting past a lot of delicate apparatus here. All the plumbing and hydraulics......'Oh,

sorry. Did you want those balls?'" (Makes radiation sound a lot more entic-
ing...) p 16

In another case discussed in the *Arizona Republic* (2003), Dwight Schaeffer was
59 when he was diagnosed with prostate cancer at the Mayo Clinic during a routine physical exam. He was otherwise healthy and had no symptoms. A biopsy
revealed that his was a fast-growing cancer so, after discussion with the urologist,
he talked to the radiologist, who helped him decide on Electron-Beam Therapy.
This was more than 12 years ago, when most non-surgical procedures were in
their infancy, but Dwight didn't like the surgery statistics, saying, "it was a risk,
but it was the right decision."

Dwight, however wasn't content to sit down and retire. He'd been an active
working adult and wanted to continue running for his own well-being and men-
tal therapy. Today, the 71-year old runs 40 to 50 miles a week, is a USA Master's
All-American in the 1500 meters for his age group (six minutes, 19 seconds) and
credits "running for being a big part of the equation that led to my recovery...as
part of a holistic approach to cancer management. The Mayo Clinic," he says,
"has always supported my efforts in that regard."

At age 60, after the E-Beam treatment was doing its job, he went back to school
and became a neuromuscular therapist, then moved to Arizona. He recommends

> "...as a prostate patient, becoming an informed patient, doing your research
> on your condition versus the options for treatment, and incorporating a holis-
> tic approach into your treatment regimen that includes diet and exercise"

Dwight's experience (and outcomes) were much different from the patient we
interviewed in the note earlier, proving once again that it is important to find the
best treatment for the circumstances a person is in, and, more importantly, spend-
ing the time to find the *best* doctor/clinic to conduct the treatment. It is apparent
that once a treatment decision has been made, it is important to find the best
"applications-doctor" to do the treatment. The one with the *most* experience who
has perfected the "art" of treatment, is the place you want to put your trust in.

It's like choosing an artist to paint your portrait; the final result will be most positive if you find the "artist" who can do the work properly. The analogy holds for

brachytherapy, external-beam, or radical prostatectomy: Do your homework; seek more than one or two opinions, then make your choice with confidence.

OTHER BOOKS WORTH READING

As Dr. Grado noted in the Forward to this text, there are very few books published by the popular press on prostate cancer, for a variety of reasons. Most books written on the subject are personal experiences, written much like a diary of events that took place when the diagnosis was positive. Most publishing houses are not interested in books, even in life and death chronicles about cancer, unless they are written by celebrities or recognized medical professionals. Thus, this *primer* probably will not be published by a big-name publisher, because it will most likely not be a big seller that makes money. That's understandable and even acceptable to the authors, as long as whoever does publish it ensures that it gets into the right people's hands: doctors, hospitals, and (most importantly) men who need to learn about prostate health and options for treatment.

There are two books, however, that are highly recommended that fall in the category of "personal experiences" of their authors, but which have lots of information about prostate health within their pages. Both are books that are published by internet companies (1stbooks.com) and are available digitally or in hard copy. A brief description follows later in this chapter (*).

A third book that is highly recommended was published by the American Cancer Society (ACS) in 1996 through Random House, Inc., and is titled simply: *PROSTATE CANCER, What Every Man—and His Family—Needs to Know*. It is an excellent book, written and edited by a team of doctors (D.G. Bostwick, G.T. MacLennan, and T.R. Larson), with input from many more in various clinics and medical treatment facilities across the U.S. (including, Dr. Gordon Grado, at that time head of Radiology at Mayo Clinic/Scottsdale, who wrote the foreward to this primer). It is an excellent book because of its descriptions, if not its current relevance to prostate cancer today (i.e. much of the technology and treatment was still in its infancy in 1996), seven plus years after it was written.

The ACS book is highly recommended (with the caveat that a significant amount of it is out-dated) for its well-written explanations of procedures and anatomical descriptions (which are *not* out-dated). It has a lot of those pictures and graphs and charts that are intentionally missing from this primer, and all those things are located in this one excellently written source. Also, as of mid-2003, it is still available from the American Cancer Society and perhaps booksellers on the Web like Amazon.com. Its just too bad that no one has edited and updated the 1996 materials in a version that more accurately reflects the current state of the art for prostate cancer treatment options.

(*)TWO BOOKS OF PERSONAL EXPERIENCES

PROSTATE CANCER BATTLE: IT'S STRICTLY YOUR DECISION is written by Professor Michael O'Hara and was published by 1st Books in 2001. It has not yet become a runaway best-seller (and it probably never will), but page for page, it has more good information and charts and diagrams than most doctor's offices. And, like this primer, it's all about providing options and written by a prostate cancer survivor with straight talk about taking control of your life.

In fact, Professor O'Hara might have provided more information than most men would want to look at. He has included copies of his PSA tests, biopsy results, MRI scans and a lot of actual written communications from his own journey that are highly enlightening. The cost of his book from the internet site is under five bucks, so for a broad perspective, you cannot beat Professor O'Hara's 225 pages of insight.

Interestingly, Professor O'Hara chose (Iodine) radiation seed treatment and in a post-script at the back of his book, he had this to say:

> "In retrospect, the only thing that would have made my road less pressured and the specific decision making process smoother would have been to have had immediate access to a book on prostate cancer like this one (his book). Then, when first appraised by my HMO physician that I had flunked my prostate biopsy, I would have been prepared to deal with the dilemma with a great deal less emotion and frustration." (pp 219)

DROP YOUR DRAWERS: Excellent Advice!

The second text that is also published by 1st Books is available in both digital and hard copy, written by Dr. Rupert Wentworth, titled *CAUGHT WITH MY PANTS DOWN (2002)* is "about Prostate Cancer, Metastatic Prostate Cancer, and more." It is highly recommended reading, because it illustrates what can happen when the chosen treatment is ineffective in stopping the spread of prostate cancer.

In particular, Dr. Wentworth went to one of the most prestigious medical clinics in America and had a radical prostatectomy performed that, he presumed, cured his cancer. Five years later, in 2000, his cancer metasticized in other parts of his body, and he commenced a journey that is today an ongoing struggle to stay alive and maintain a good quality of life in the process.

Both these books are personal journeys that echo what this text is about; the more information a man can get about prostate treatment options, the better he will be able to reduce the risk factors and choose a successful treatment. We highly recommend both the Wentworth and O'Hara books, together with the ACS book, for a complete understanding of prostate cancer. With those three books, plus this text and access to the internet sites recommended in Chapter 5 of this Primer, you have the most up-to-date decision-making tools available at this point in time (2004) on prostate cancer.

FACING CHOICES: Get More Opinions

Just as in our discussion earlier in this chapter, and in the books recommended above, Wentworth, O'Hara, Ackerman and Schaeffer were all faced with treatment choices. While there may be fewer high-percentage treatment types than six or eight that are candidates, the three *proven* prostate cancer-killer therapies with the highest probability of success are Radical Prostatectomy, External-Beam Radiation (E-Beam), and Brachytherapy. Each therapy has its advantages and disadvantages, so the choice a man makes depends on his own individual (physical) situation. The good news, however, is that information is more and more available on how to make choices, and your continued best health options are dependent on acquiring and using that information.

A THIRD BOOK FROM THE NATIONAL PROSTATE CANCER COALITION

Normally, we would not recommend books or texts we have not reviewed, but the National Prostate Cancer Coalition in Washington, D.C. has a lot of good advice and a web site (www.pcacoalition.org) where they regularly update prostate cancer information and they have a book available that is a bit of a different perspective that we recommend checking out. The book is written by the wife of a gentleman that NPCA says is "the nation's leading lay expert on prostate cancer." (Their words, not ours.)

The reason we recommend this book is because it is written by a diagnosed man's wife, and therefore offers advice and words of encouragement to other wives and *significant other's* going through the prostate cancer experience with their partners, which is a point-of-view no other written materials seem to take. The author, (wife) Desiree Lyon Howe, is also a board member of the NPCC and that probably has something to do with their endorsement of her book, but we think it's worth checking out, especially for the "partners" of men diagnosed with this disease.

HUNDREDS OF MORE "PERSONAL" WRITINGS

As noted earlier, there are hundreds of articles and papers written by diagnosed men which appear in magazines and medical references. The few we have chosen to mention here are, however, ones we considered to be the best range of information for the newly diagnosed man who needs to gather as much information as possible in as short a time as possible. Urologists and prostate cancer specialists will also have a lot of literature reference materials, but just as with the advice to seek out second and third opinions on your specific problem, we recommend seeking as many different books, magazines and sources of printed materials on the problem also.

While you will find differing opinions and sometimes conflicting interpretations of the same data, you owe it to yourself (and your significant other) to sift and sort the information and decide what *you* need to do for your own peace of mind; not your doctors! S/he will not be the one living with the consequences of the treatment you choose, so be diligent and open-minded. And, above all else, ask questions and be persistent. It's *your* life!

3

INTRODUCTION

It is commonly understood that prostate cancer is *usually* very slow growing cancer. (emphasis on *usually*) But if you are diagnosed with prostate cancer, what does that mean? Do you have *years* to deal with it? Do you have *months*? Or should you be dealing with it as soon as possible, even though it may be slow growing—it could still be dangerous, so shouldn't you do something as quickly as possible?

The answer to these questions, at least with today's medical knowledge of the subject, is "it depends." There are so many variables to consider when trying to decide what the time frame is for taking a treatment action that it is difficult to give a checksheet of options and a timeline that meets every individual's situation.

SECOND AND THIRD OPINIONS: Absolutely, *Positively* Required!

Recently, the American Association of Retired People (AARP) monthly newsletter/bulletin (February, 2003) reported on the importance of getting second and third opinions for critical diagnosis. In the article, several cancer experts and clinical studies were quoted, one notably relevant for prostate cancer. Professor Jerome Groopman, M.D. at the Medical School at Harvard University, has even written a book on the importance of second opinions (*Second Opinions,* Penquin USA, 2001). He quotes Ernest Rosenbaum, M.D. who is in Clinical medicine at Stanford University, who says,

> "…the question is not why you should get a second opinion, but why would you not? There is no scientific downside."

Further, Groopman and Rosenbaum point out that most doctors *encourage* patients to seek out a second opinion because they need to feel comfortable with their own diagnostics. Groopman notes that doctors who do not welcome a second opinion should serve as a red flag; something is wrong here.

Dr. Groopman notes

> "…if your father had prostate cancer, he was probably told it had to be removed surgically and that was that. Today, a biopsy determines the stage of the cancer—and the recommended treatment can absolutely change as a result of subtle differences that may only be detected through a second opinion."

That's good advice, and comes from years of diagnosing and treating varying types of cancer. Dr Groopman and Dr. Rosenblum, who chairs the Department of Pathology at Memorial Sloan-Kettering Cancer Center in New York City, have been analyzing tumors for a combined total of more than 50 years. They point out that

> "…analyzing even the rarest tumors is second nature to a pathologist in a specialized referral center because we look at so many cases."

Further, the technology in medicine diagnostics is changing so fast that (prostate) cancer solutions and treatment options are increasing at an exponential rate. The AARP article lists ways to get the most from a second opinion:

GETTING THE MOST FROM SECOND (AND THIRD) OPINIONS
(from Stanford University's Dr. Rosenbaum):

*Tell your doctor you want another review *and* enlist his help. "It's a terrible mistake to go behind your doctors back for a second opinion because you're afraid he'll be mad at you."

*Take notes during the second opinion interview, or even better, tape it, even if you're accompanied by a relative or friend. This lets you review the information at your own pace.

*If your health plan won't cover a second opinion, pay for one yourself if at all possible. (After all, it may be your life that hangs in the balance.)

*Use organizations such as the American Heart Association, the American Cancer Society and the National Cancer Institute for information and referral sources. The Richard and Annette Bloch Cancer Foundation (www. blastcancer.org) offers a list of major cancer referral centers throughout the country.

*Approach second (and third) opinions on the Internet with extreme caution. Thousands of websites claim to offer opinions by qualified doctors, and it's difficult to detect the quacks.

*If your first and second doctors don't agree, get a third opinion (or more!). Medicare and many private health plans pay.

(Web sites you need to know and phone numbers where you can contact the experts: American Heart Association, www.americanheart.org or Ph (800)-242-8721; the American Cancer Society, www.cancer.org or (800)-227-2345; the National Cancer Institute, www.nci.nih. Also, see the web sites listed in Chapter Four for more information on prostate cancer.)

YOUR FUTURE, YOUR LIFE: Taking Responsibility

As a summary to this chapter, we reiterate that a man faced with the possibility of prostate cancer (right from the first DRE that the GP conducts as a part of a routine physical exam) needs to seek out *more than* one opinion on 1) selection of biopsy; 2) selecting the right urologist (if a biopsy is to be performed); 3) understanding the many treatment options (if biopsy results are positive) or, 4) understanding what to do if biopsy results are "negative." (Sometimes this finding can be as perplexing to the man having nighttime symptoms as a positive finding.)

The key for any man embarking on this prostate cancer journey is obviously to get second, and even more opinions. At the very least, decisions of this magnitude will determine how much longer you may live (with or without cancer) and the quality of your life from this day forward. All those variables and uncertainties require strategic decision-making, utilizing the best medical data and doctors' opinions available. It's your responsibility to yourself and to your loved ones. Seek more opinions!

P.S. WHAT ABOUT YOUR FAMILY?

We have talked a lot about getting second opinions (and third, fourth or more!) and how important it is for the man who's going through the "process" of prostate treatment research and decision-making. What we haven't discussed is for the man who is married or who has a "significant other" who is part of his life, she will have just as many fears and questions that need answers, and sometimes more! The impact to the "family" of cancer treatment choice cannot be understated, and a man must deal with those realities upfront.

Fortunately, there are places where information can be obtained to help the whole family deal with prostate cancer. In the ACS book recommended earlier, an entire chapter is devoted to helping find support for the entire family. Among other information, there are support groups for cancer of all types and varieties, but there are support groups for prostate cancer specifically, which are listed and detailed in the ACS chapter. However, for our contribution in this primer, we will mention only one, called "US TOO."

US TOO was founded in 1990 and is a national organization which is administered by (volunteer) prostate cancer survivors. It has more than 400 chapters with 60,000 members and over 100,000 family members represented throughout the world with headquarters at 930 N. York Road, Suite 50; Hinsdale, IL 60521 and a toll free phone: 800-808-7866. (If those address and phone numbers have changed, check the internet for updated information at www.ustoo. com/chapters.)

In summary, men need to realize that the impact of prostate problems affects the family, also, and that they are not alone when it comes to seeking help. Through organizations like US TOO, families can find they are not alone; help is only a click away.

4

In this chapter, you will learn about…

Rethinking Treatment Options: The Mayo Clinic Study

When Should Men start PSA screening?

Discussing Cancer Screening With Doctors

MAYO CLINIC STUDIES: Rethinking Radiation Treatment Options

A recent Mayo Clinic study by Dr. O.K. McDonald and Dr. Steven Schild (Mayo Clinic, 2003) of men who have had a reoccurrence of cancer after a prostatectomy was conducted in Scottsdale, Arizona focused on men whose PSA levels rose after surgery, up to five years later. The results showed, among other things, that 20% of men whose prostates were removed have their PSA levels rise, indicating that cancer has come back.

In the Mayo study, 60 men with elevated PSA levels were given radiation treatments over seven weeks at the site where the prostate was removed. They followed the treated men, and after 5 years half the men treated with radiation are free of cancer, with those men who received higher radiation doses doing better than those treated with lower doses.

In discussing the conclusions of the study at the Chicago meeting of the American Society of Clinical Oncology (May, 2003), Dr., Schild noted that when primary care providers and urologists send someone for radiation treatment, it's better to send them earlier than later. "Now that we know that men who have a return of cancer after a prostatectomy should be treated with higher dosages of radiation to improve chances for a cure."

The priority treatment at Mayo Clinic has historically been radical prostatectamy for most cancer patients, no matter what Gleason Scores indicate. It appears, on the basis of this study, the Mayo Clinic oncologists, urologists, and prostate specialists are now taking a second look at that policy, perhaps to looking at brachytherapy and Electron-Beam treatment before recommending radical prostatectomy as the first priority.

PSA SCREENING: What Age to Start?

In keeping with our concern about younger men (i.e. we discussed this earlier in Chapter 2), it's been shown that GP's are beginning to take more seriously the DRE in routine physical exams. There is a sharper awareness in the general medical community that PSA results should be *routinely* requested in blood work for physical examinations, although there is some evidence that insurance companies are balking at paying for this test in men under the age of 50 without justification on a case-by-case basis.

There is also a growing concern, among the GP community at least, that men who have symptoms of prostate problems should be more closely observed and followed and sent to urologists for evaluation, even when PSA results are low. It isn't clear if the impetus for this follow-up is concern about malpractice or if its because the medical community has noticed a trend toward younger men being diagnosed with prostate cancer (and not just BPH, as had previously been assumed). But the medical community in general has become more sensitive to cancer as more and more work has been done on the diagnostic side of medicine. The results are more important for men; more attention is now being focused on prostate cancer than at anytime in history.

The consensus of doctors involved in men's health now appears to be directed toward taking a hard look at PSA results on physical exams that are otherwise routine. The picture we need to paint now is that men of every age should be as knowledgeable about what PSA means (i.e. how good an indicator it is or is not) as they can be. If this book accomplishes nothing else, that should be one issue that gets clearly defined. PSA is the best indicator *at this point in time* (emphasis added!) of the potential for prostate cancer to be present. It is not, however, infallible, and numerical values assigned to it are debated by specialists across the medical professions. Is a result of 2.9 different from 2.5? Should you be concerned if PSA results are greater than _____. (Fill in a number; there will be some who say "yes" and some who say "no.") What is important to know is that there should be a follow-up if the numerical value consistently rises from blood tests taken 3 or 4 times over as many months. That "trend" rise indicates the possibility that something is going on and a urologist needs to evaluate your options.

Whether or not a biopsy should be conducted under that circumstance is, of course, a matter of agreement between you and your doctor. Second opinions are encouraged to get consensus, but generally a rising PSA (with values greater than 3.5) probably should result in a biopsy. Even then, understand the biopsy procedure and the risks that procedure subjects you to before selecting the doctor to conduct it. (Read Chapters One and Three again!)

Some clinics and prostate doctors look at the PSA results in age increments. For instance, for men who have PSA results less than 3.0, most will say there's nothing to worry about, but to re-test in 2 to 6 months to see if it increases. For men bracketed in the age group 40 to 50, some will say a PSA of less than 3.0 is OK, while for men age 50 to 60 they might say a PSA score of up to 4.0 is OK. For men 50 to 60, they might say a PSA up to 5.0 is OK and for men 60 to 70, they might say a PSA of up to 6.0 would be OK, prescribing "watch and wait" for each of those age brackets and PSA scores. For men over 70, they may say "don't worry until the PSA reaches greater than, say, 6.5, and even then, re-testing every 3 months to see if there is a trend might be the prognosis.

It is not our recommendation, however, to interpret PSA numbers by a sliding scale in age brackets. Our research findings for this primer seems to show consistent agreement with the idea that PSA scores greater than 3.0 for *any* age should be followed with re-testing over a six month period. The exception might be for men overage 70 or 75, where higher PSA scores might require retesting only every 6 months, to see if a trend is developing. Even then, it may be questionable to recommend "treatment" for the man who has other more serious medical conditions. Again, this is the place for men to get second and third opinions before deciding to take any sort of action.

The fact that more and more doctors are concerned about accurately communicating the pros and cons of prostate health is supported in the literature. More clinics and hospitals are making prostate information available now than ever before. But doctors who treat and diagnose prostate problems are not any more forthcoming than they ever have been, and men need to understand how to get answers *before* they decide on a specific treatment regime, especially where cancer has been diagnosed. Thus at the end of this chapter we have provided some sources of information where a better understanding of prostate functions, treatments, and side-effects can be obtained.

DISCUSSING CANCER SCREENING WITH DOCTORS

Because there is a renewed emphasis within the medical community on making sure that prostate cancer is diagnosed in its earliest stages, there are differing opinions on what the diagnostic steps should be. For patients who come to the GP with symptoms, there is an almost universal tendency for recommending follow-up with a urologist. (Here is where the "communications" begin to break down, for the patient and we talk about that problem here). For the routine physical exam that shows PSA abnormalities or DRE deviation of the prostate gland, we find that whatever recommendation is made to the patient is related to how old the examining physician is and how long he or she has been in practice! Most of this "finding" is based on anecdotal or hearsay from conversations with patients, but the information is valuable for the newly concerned man going for recommendations.

INFORMATION SOURCES

The advent of the World Wide Web (Internet) has provided anyone who has access to a computer, anywhere in the world, access to data and information that was never before possible. Gone are the days when the only way to learn about an unfamiliar topic or subject was to go to a city or college library, use the card catalog and/or consult the librarian to conduct a research of the literature that took days or even weeks. Even then, obtaining even half of the information requested was hit or miss, depending upon how capable the research assistant was and how big the library capability was to "cover the globe."

Today, there are internet access kiosks at coffee shops and in the smallest of town libraries and easy "how to" guides to make a novice computer hacker an expert at finding information. For purposes of this book, we have included some of the sites (i.e. even this list will lead to more sites that are linked to these) that may prove useful to the interested researcher specific to prostate cancer information.

One note of caution: the internet sites come and go with more being added daily to the World Wide Web. Therefore, the sites noted here are not a comprehensive list and, as of late 2003, represents only a few that are now available. So when (and if) you go to the internet, you can query sites like, "www.askjeeves.com" or "www.google.com" by searching for the key words, such as "brachytherapy" or "prostate," or any combination of words related to the topic. What those sites will do is "connect" you to sites that have those words or phrases as a partial subject for their site. After searching for a while, you will find that you begin to get repeated site names more and more frequently as they seem to "link together." Thus at that point you will probably want to begin getting into the sites that you think give you the information you are looking for and conclude your mission of searching for new sites.

In total, however, you will find conflicting advice and you will need to think for yourself, sound out your thoughts with your doctor(s) and talk to other men who have the same problem to be sure you can make decisions about your own situation. The key is, however, *be informed* and don't accept *one* opinion from *one* doctor. It's *your* prostate! It's *your* health! And, it's *your* responsibility to yourself to get the best advice and information you can.

WORLD WIDE WEB SITES

A simple search on the Web by typing in google.com might yield a hundred or more sites that have something to offer related to "Prostate Cancer Treatment" if those three words are typed in and the "search" button is clicked. The list below provides just a few that come up when such a search is initiated; some will be better than others but only a few will answer *your* particular questions about *your* situation:

WWW.CMHPROSTATE.COM
WWW.KRONGRAD-UROLOGY.COM
WWW.YOUNGAGAIN.COM
WWW.CTRCCANCERTRIALS.COM
WWW.CANCERFACTS.COM
WWW.MENSHEALTHTECH.COM

WWW.AVMAZON.COM/BETTER-PROSTATE
WWW.MALECARE.COM
WWW.NLM.NIH.GOV/MEDLINEPLUS/PROSTATECANCER
WWW.VIADUR.COM/
WWW.PCACOALITION.ORG
WWW.PROSTATE.COM/
WWW.HENRYFORD.COM
WWW.ICHTIPT.COM
WWW.CMHPROSTATE.COM
WWW.YOUNGAGAIN2000.COM
WWW.ISSELS.COM
WWW.NUTRITION200.COM
WWW.SITOSTEROL-SAW-PALMENTO-PROSTATITIS-
TREATMENT.COM
WWW.CANADAPHARMACY.COM
WWW.DRCATALONA.COM
WWW.MSKCC.ORG/MSKCC
WWW.CANCER.GOV
WWW.4NPCC.ORG
HTTP://UROLOGY.JHU.EDU

SUMMARY: Men of All Ages: Take Charge!

We summarize this chapter with an admonishment (risking redundancy) that men need to be better informed about their prostate health and recommend that they seek out every source of information they can find. This would be essential not only for men who are just beginning to have prostate symptoms, but also for men who have never had reason to be concerned. The message is this: get a PSA every year, together with an annual physical exam, starting at age 40!

The cost for a physical exam, even if you must pay for it out-of-pocket, is cheap when compared with finding a problem when it's too late to treat it. Prostate cancer is treatable and curable—if it's caught in the early stages. Ordinary physical examinations which include a PSA in the blood screen will pay dividends in the cost-benefit analysis.

The choices you have if and when results show cause for concern are expanding every day for most men's diseases, and especially in cancers like prostate and colon; early diagnosis is essential to living a long and healthy life. In order to do this right, men absolutely *must* be proactive and take charge of their physical conditions. Take yearly exams; develop a good rapport with your GP, and communicate! It's *your* life; live it!

5

INTRODUCTION

"Prevention" has become a much used and abused word in medicine today, but it really is the best way to ensure that people live a lifestyle today that recognizes that what they eat and how they exercise (or don't) can have significant benefits in the prevention of disease in the future. Some physicians believe that this is the only way, in fact, to give the body the best opportunity to prevent diseases—including cancer—from starting. Statistics on life and death in the 21st century appear to bear that out: In 1900, the average baby born could expect to live 47.3 years, while in 2000, life expectancy had risen to 76.9 years. According to the National Center for Health Statistics (September, 2002), drops in death rates at every stage of life and for most diseases is occurring nationwide. Even with the introduction of killer diseases, such as AIDS, preventative life-style choices such as reduced smoking and preventative medical intervention (i.e. technology) has had a dramatic effect on increased life expectancy.

Interestingly, mortality among adults ages 45 to 64 fell by nearly 50 percent between 1950 and 2000, including drops in heart disease, strokes and injuries. But cancer is still the leading cause of death in this group, although the rates rose until 1980, when they began to drop slowly. Just as puzzling is the fact that while cancer rates have been falling since 1980, prostate cancer rates have risen over that same period. Thus statistics must always be compared and applied with a note of caution: Prostate cancer is still on the rise, and men need to understand what their risk factors are *before* making lifestyle choices.

The word "disease" is made up of two terms: "dis" and "ease," so that the noun "disease" can virtually be used to describe a plethora of maladies. That includes "cancer," of course, and any discussion of cancer should include the ways we believe that "prevention" of the disease can at least be enhanced.

In this discussion, we recognize that the jury is still out on what eating properly and exercising regularly actually contributes to *prevention*, particularly as it applies to cancer prevention. In the case of prostate cancer, this is even more obscure, because little is yet known about what causes cancer cells to suddenly begin multiplying in the gland. If we knew, we might be able to say what "preventative" measures are absolutely certain to prevent prostate cancer. But we don't know. Thus in this chapter, we explore what medical and preventative measures we believe will provide better circumstances for prevention of cancer (both general cancer in the body, as well as prostate cancer specifically).

It will be controversial once more, whenever the term "alternative medicine" is used, but such controversy is healthy, and we encourage discussion and debate on the use of alternative therapies. It is vitally important that we provide you with as much information as possible on the ways in which you might live a healthy and long life.

DO'S AND DON'TS: A Brief Review of Food Choices

Nutritionists and herbalists have a plethora of "foods" that have been promoted over the years for making up a healthy diet. Unfortunately, each practicioner seems to have favorite "foods" they like or dislike, and they are not all in agreement. In our concern to find "science-based" recommendations for this text, we have provided only those cancer-avoidance "foods" which have some scientifically validated data behind them.

As noted in the Introduction to this text, we still don't know what triggers prostate cancer tumors to grow, so we cannot say with certainty which "foods" to eat or to avoid to prevent prostate cancer. In fact, no one really knows for sure if food, in fact, has anything at all to do with prostate cancer. But nutrition science and herbal practice over the past 3000 years has given us a fairly good idea of what "foods" are more healthy and what "foods" generally cause more morbidity in the general population. It is this body of "food" science that we take our recommendations from and hope you will experiment with your own "recipes" to find out what works best for *your* body.

As noted before, Dr. Larry Clapp (*Prostate Health in 90 Days*, 2000), has written and published widely about the *correct* (*his* opinion) foods for both general health and cancer prevention. He notes that most Americans don't even come close to eating a healthy diet, preferring the four food groups beginning with the letter "f" instead: *fried* food, *fast* food, *frozen* food, and *fun* food (candy). (pp 111).

As our life styles have evolved into hectic scheduling marathons, mealtime has been sacrificed in the interest of stuffing it in before and after school activities, weekend sports, music lessons and road trips to see or play activities that almost demand fast food stops instead of home-cooked meals. It may be that if we did nothing else in the way of deciding what "foods" we should and shouldn't be eating, we could have a great impact on reducing prostate (and other) cancer simply by giving up all those hectic and stressful activities that have taken us away from family meals at home. No one, however, has studied this possibility, so we are left with speculating about what foods—given our hectic life style choices—should and shouldn't be in our diet.

FOODS AND SCIENCE

"Cows milk is for cows." That's a quote you won't see in the American Dairy Association literature, but since we know so much about dairy products and their negative effects on the human body, milk is one of those "foods" that is on the list of bad things you should not be consuming. And it's not just on a few lists; it's on most nutritionist's, dietician's, naturopath's and other professional's who see diet as one key to a healthy life. About the only medical professionals that think milk and milk products are OK for consumption are pediatricians who still refuse to look at the scientific evidence. The fact that a significant percentage of babies reject cow's milk (and must be fed lactose intolerance medicine or soy-based substitutes) should be enough evidence that, "cow's milk is (truly) for cows," and not humans.

Dairy products, especially cheese-based foods which happen to be almost a "sta-ple" in our hectic fast-food life style (i.e. pizza and cheese-filled snack foods, cheese burgers and cheese-based Mexican food have become the best selling fast foods in the U.S.) make this diet staple a key player in the general population. By the way, according to Dr. Clapp (2000), studies have shown a high correlation between prostate cancer and dairy product consumption, so for our purposes, eliminating dairy products in men's diets should be considered a priority.

LIFESTYLE CHOICES: Living A Healthy Life

In this section we discuss some of the studies and literature that show promise for "prevention" of disease (primarily for cancer of the prostate). By illustrating where herbal remedies and Chinese medicines have been successful, we segue into cancer prevention through the use of these same techniques.

ALTERNATIVE MEDICINE AND TREATMENT TECHNIQUES

In recent times, the medical community has begun to embrace the use of hereto-fore unhearlded forms of treatment for all sorts of maladies. Notable among his peers, Dr. Andrew Weil at the University of Arizona Medical Center has been leading the way with incorporation of alternative medical techniques in his traditional practice. In addition, Dr. Dharma Singh Khalsa has also utilized "meditation for medicine" techniques to help patients in the clinical setting.

ONCE AGAIN: Get More Than One Opinion

In keeping with our intent to be a "primer" of information about male prostate disease(s) in general, and cancer of the prostate gland in particular, it should be painfully obvious that there is as much unknown as there is "known" about prostate cancer. While that is obvious in the literature, the lay-public is mostly not aware that doctors (and medical community professionals in general) are not accustomed to telling their patients that they don't have all the answers. But it is true. The public has placed medical professionals on the elite pedestal for so long that it's almost taken for granted that they are experts in every facet of medicine, even if they only profess to be specialists in one area of medical practice.

Interestingly, doctors (of all types) are allowed to "practice" their art, just as lawyers are allowed to "practice" law. Yet we members of the lay-public (who become their patients and clients) are expected to fully trust their words, as though they are infallible diagnosticians. Thus if we allow ourselves to step back and take a deep breath whenever we are faced with diagnostics and prognostication from or about a serious medical condition, we allow ourselves to make choices such as seeking out second and third opinions before we choose a therapy or treatment for the malady that has been diagnosed. Men need to remember this before placing their blind faith in one doctor's opinion. Keep repeating: get another opinion! (And, another…and, another…etc.)

As noted earlier in this text, that is one of the most common problems with men when they are diagnosed with (prostate) cancer; they ask the doctor, "What's my choice for treatment?" and make the implicit assumption that this professional's opinion is infallible, since s/he has several years of medical school and years of experience to back it up. It is no different with trying to utilize any particular alternative medicine or alternative treatment; *there are no experts,* even among the "doctors" and other "medical professionals" that endorse a particular alternative treatment method.

DON'T ASK; DON'T TELL

Recently, the Newsletter from *Lets Talk Health* 2003, (www.letstalkhealth.com) featured an interview with several medical doctors on the general subject of prescription and alternative medications and pharmaceutical industry costs. Dr. Jerry Avorn, a research physician at Harvard Medical School, said it best about knowing what medications to prescribe.

> "If patients were aware of the limitations that all of us physicians have in terms of what we know and what we wish we knew and what we don't know, they would be more scared than they are at present. Always wait a year before prescribing a new drug, and if it is for a family member, wait five years! We really don't know as much as we would like to know about a drug until it's been around for awhile…"

So, now you've heard it from the most prestigious of medical schools; prescription medications are a crap-shoot and you need to be talking to your doctor *and* your pharmacist to get all the right information.

PREVENTION AND ALTERNATIVE MEDICINE

Private herbal supply companies of all varieties have products purporting to be "the answer" to making your prostate healthy and/or preventing prostate cancer from occurring. Some purveyors provide charts and facts to back up their products. Since there is little scientific proof for such claims, it's "buyer beware." But there are "good sense" precautions that can be taken, and the use of the proper herbal products are among the best.

Researchers at the National Cancer Institute report that a diet with lots of vegetables from the allium food group—which includes garlic, shallots and onions—reduces the risk of prostate cancer by about half. The normal Chinese diet includes hearty servings of these vegetables. and previous studies have supported the general finding that eating vegetables is a good thing.

In this study which appeared in the *Journal of the National Cancer Institute*, 238 men with known prostate cancer and 471 men (thought to be) free of the disease were interviewed. All the men in the study were residents of Shanghai, China and were asked how frequently they ate 122 food items.

The results showed that those who ate more than a third of an ounce a day from the allium food group were about 50 percent *less* likely to have prostate cancer than those who ate less of the foods. The conclusions still need to be replicated in further studies to be sure the results are statistically significant, but the researchers believe—based on previous confirmatory research findings—that further research will bear out the fact that eating vegetables like scallions, onions, and garlic is a prostate-cancer-preventative.

Other researchers at the Fred Hutchinson Cancer Research Center in Seattle confirmed that the results supports findings in some of their own studies; garlic and onions may be bad for your breath, but they are good for your prostate! But for the record, chlorophyll-coated garlic tablets are available that don't give you garlic breath!

LOOKING FOR SCIENCE: Ask the Scientists!

There are lots of reports in the papers these days about cancer and the relationship of foods we eat to both prevention and cures. Its not the purpose of this book to throw a lot of contradictory information out and confuse the issue, so in the interest of being as"scientific" as possible, we've chosen to use the National Cancer Institute research and its recommendations to summarize this controversial subject.

Here's the bottom line from NCI:

1.) Thirty percent or more cancers are linked to the foods we eat. Over generations, the move from a diet high in plant-based foods to one significantly lower in plant foods may be one reason for higher rates of cancer.

2.) Vegetables, fruits, and whole grains contain essential vitamins and minerals, as well as hundreds of phytochemicals that may protect against cancer and other chronic diseases such as heart disease.

3.) Over 200 studies worldwide clearly show that a plant-rich diet lowers the risk of numerous cancers. The key to this protection may be the way nutrients and phytochemicals in foods work together against cancer. NCI believes you can signifi-cantly lower your risk of getting cancer by regularly eating certain foods and avoiding others.

4.) Reduced cancer risk can come from avoidance and reduction of consumption of fats, especially animal fats, red meat, grilled or overcooked meats, pickled and salt-cured meats, and those in which aflatoxins are present. In particular, evidence suggests that a diet high in fats may be linked to an increased risk of several cancers, prostate cancer included, while red meats are linked to an increased risk of colon and prostate cancer.

5.) Reducing intake of (animal) fats and increasing fiber in the diet significantly reduces risk of cancer. Check the American Cancer Society and/or National Cancer Institute web sites for more information.

VITAMINS AND HERBS: Not a Substitute

We hear a lot these days about taking supplements; calcium, vitamin A, B, C, E, B-12, beta-carotene, antioxidants, free radical scavengers, etc. seem to be the subject of articles in the media every day. What is usually not apparent is that advice given about the value of taking these various and assorted "supplements" almost lulls the reader into believing that, "popping a few daily vitamins will substitute for not eating right!"

Nothing could be further from the truth. Thus for our purposes here, there are some basic truths we need to state: supplemental vitamins may be essential for most people because most of us do not eat properly and tend not to get the daily ration of what the experts think is essential. But—and it is a very BIG "but," supplements are not a substitute for eating the proper diet, especially the proper foods that lower cancer risk (as noted before in this chapter).

Most nutritionists, and indeed most physicians who know the value of foods in preventive medicine, agree that there are 13 essential nutrients which the body cannot make in adequate amounts for the body's daily needs, let alone in amounts that are considered *cancer risk preventative.*

In addition, there are others—perhaps as many as 17 or 18—that are only stored in the body for a short time before they "wash out" so they need replenishment more often, and supplements can provide those.

HERBS AND HERBALS

There is a difference in vitamins and herbs, even though the mass media seems to lump the two into the same class of "supplemental health aids." The distinction may be subtle; many vitamins are actually made of herbal ingredients. However, for our purposes it is important that men facing dietary decisions to combat prostate cancer understand the distinction. Vitamins can be thought of as, classically, those things that the USDA says our bodies require. We see these in advertisements as "recommended Daily Dose" for Vitamin B, Vitamin C, Vitamin E; etc., etc.

Herbs may also be a "vitamin" or be an ingredient in a particular vitamin complex, but they may also be considered "food" that the body uses to enhance overall health or health of particular organs. Just as Vitamin C is required for healthy bones and teeth, an herb like "saw palmetto" has been used both as a preventive and corrective for prostate problems. By building the thyroid to control the operation of glands, saw palmetto helps overcome such men's health problems as enlarged prostate, underdeveloped testicles, sterility and impotence.

According to *Nature's Field Distributor's Newsletter* (March/April 1999), saw palmetto has been shown in studies in Europe to be more effective for BPH sufferers than the drug (proscar), most often recommended to relieve this condition. (See also *Potter's New Encyclopedia of Botanical Drugs and Preparations* by R.C. Wrens; Essex, England; C.W. Daniel Company Limited, 1985).

Other BPH herbals include combinations of horsetail herb, black cohosh root, uva ursi leaves, licorice root, kelp plant, capsicum fruit, golden seal root, and ginger root. Other herbs that have been shown in studies to help overcome prostate problems include stinging nettle (which does not sting when its taken in dried form), and gotu kola (hydrocotyle asiatica), which is another herbal preparation that can be used for enlarged prostate. Many prostate-specific herbal combinations are, in fact, available from stores and naturopathic clinics that specialize in glandular problem prevention and/or cancer treatment.

An excellent source of information on herbs and supplements and their use for cancer treatment and cancer prevention is *Miracle Cures,* written by Jean Carper and published by Harper-Collins in 1997. It is still in print and still referenced in medical clinics for prostate health advice. It has one whole chapter devoted to prostate health by using herbs and supplements and includes documentation of the studies which support the findings.

Of course so-called case studies have been used in other papers and books about the "miracle cure of the month," but Carper's book provides documentation and reports on controlled studies to support most of her case studies. For example, she cites vitamin studies conducted at the University of Virginia and selenium studies at the University of Arizona, among others, in showing the success of dietary changes in eradicating cancer.

In addition, there are studies conducted by Dr. Keith Block at the Cancer Institute in Chicago that have shown success in cancer treatment in a variety of patients. The evidence is mounting; herbs and supplements are being used with conventional cancer therapies to increase success and decrease side effects.

WATERMELON: Sweet Lycopene

Tomatoes get the headlines for their protective effect against prostate cancer, but "ounce for ounce, watermelon contains 40% more of the active cancer-fighting compound lycopene than tomatoes," according to Dr. David Kiefer, a fellow in the University of Arizona's Program in Integrative Medicine. Kiefer is a researcher in the program headed by alternative medicine guru Andrew Weil, M.D., and says that their studies show that not only is lycopene crucial in overall prostate health. Kiefer suggests that "other studies are showing that it may block the plaque buildup in arteries that can lead to heart attack, and it may offset some of the cellular damage and aging effects that lead to Alzheimer's, Parkinson's, and arthritis." (AARP, Sept/Oct 2003)

VITAMINS SHOWN IN STUDIES TO REDUCE PROSTATE CANCER RISK

There have been several studies that have shown that certain vitamins reduce cancer risk, and reports from NCI, ACS, and some like the London Hospital research have shown promise for prostate cancer specifically. The vitamin which has shown the most promise and for which there seems to be the most scientific evidence is Vitamin E. In studies cited by Richard Harkness, Steven Bratman and David Kroll in *The Natural Pharmacist* (also available on www.TNP.com on the internet), a 1998 study in Finland of more than 36,000 adults found that a diet low in vitamin E increased overall cancer risk by 50%!

They also cited a study of 11,178 elderly individuals who reported taking vitamin E had an overall 59% reduction in cancer deaths. Even after adjusting the data for alcohol use, smoking history, aspirin use and other medical conditions, the results were the same. The researchers concluded that vitamin E supplements could also help prevent death from heart disease in this same study.

In a study of 29,000 male smokers in Finland who took supplements of either 50 mg of vitamin E, 20 mg of betacarotene, both or a placebo daily for 5 to 8 years, there was a 32% lower incidence of prostate cancer and 41% fewer prostate cancer deaths. They also reported, surprisingly, that the positive results came soon after the start of supplementation and have concluded that the vitamin E might block the progression of the slow-growing prostate cancer cells (although this conclusion is not supported by the study itself).

They have also speculated that because this study was aimed at looking at smokers and the impact of vitamin E on lung cancer, it is reasonable to think that vitamin E might work even better on non-smokers. Studies are underway currently to replicate the results.

SUMMARIZING SCIENCE

Studies are accumulating in reputable institutions that show that what we eat may have a major role to play in cancer prevention and cancer cure. Specific studies have been cited by the National Cancer Institute (NCI) and the American Cancer Institute (ACI) and at private research centers in the U.S. and Europe which show that the evidence supporting the role of food and nutrients (i.e. supplements) for cancer prevention is growing.

New research at traditional medical institutions where non-traditional medicine is playing a significant role is breaking ground every day. Andrew Weil at the University of Arizona Medical Center, prostate cancer research at Cedars Sinai in Los Angeles supported by the Michael Milken Foundation, NCI-funded prostate research at the Cleveland Institute and the J. Hayden Fry Center for Prostate Cancer Research at the University of Iowa (U of I) are just a few of the newest efforts to find preventative techniques and treatments for prostate cancer.

Recently, the National Institute of Health awarded the U of I $2.5 million to study if phytotherapy is effective in treating the enlarged prostate (i.e. BPH). There are actually 10 institutions nationwide participating in the Complimentary and Alternative Medicines for Urology Symptoms study, so we are hopeful that one of the study spin-offs will show the validity of using phytotherapy (i.e. the use of plant extracts) for prostate cancer, too.

With the national effort toward curing cancers of all types, and the encouraging new research efforts utilizing diet and supplement research for prostate cancer prevention, we can be optimistic that prostate cancer can one day be eradicated. Until that time comes, diet and nutrition certainly needs to be a part of every man's risk reduction plan because if its not a part of the solution, diet is most certainly a part of the problem.

REALITY: Drugs Are Big Business

You've seen the statistics, and every day in TV news and in the newspapers we are bombarded with advertising by pharmaceutical companies about specific drugs they are claiming you cannot live without. "Ask your doctor," they all say, implying that your doctor is going to endorse their prescription medication for you. How much more confidence could you have that those medical professionals once again have your best interests at heart? Little wonder that it's difficult to get good research (data) on alternative medicines when main stream drug companies exert such control over funding.

But realize that consumers spent $90 billion more on prescription drugs in 2001 than they did five years before, in 1996! "Sure," you say, "but drug companies need to get their research investment back for the millions they spent developing those great drugs." But that's before you realize that the drug industry spent $15 billion in 2001 in advertising to get you to ask for particular drugs and to get doctors to prescribe them! Does all this paint a picture of collusion between the medical practicioners and drug companies, with *you* playing the role of guinea pig in the middle? And who's paying for it? You guessed it! We guinea pigs!

Dr. Drummond Rennie is an editor at the *Journal of the American Medical Association* (JAMA) who's not afraid to state the obvious. He says researchers who are critical of the establishment get attacked all the time. "I believe" he's quoted on www.letstalkhealth.com (July, 2003) as saying, "that drug companies are intent on keeping the consumer on drugs for the simple requirement of profit."

And that's from the JAMA, one of the most quoted and prestigious of medical journals of research in the world. Is it any wonder that *herbal* medications get such bad press?

RUNNING FROM CANCER: Walking May Be As Good

In the May, 2003 edition of *Energy Times* (pp 70), studies by the UCLA Jonsson Cancer Center and Department of Physiological Science have found that a strict walking regimen, along with a high-fiber, low fat diet can slow the growth of prostate cancer cells by up to 30%. According to William Aronson, the senior study author, the study strongly suggests that a low-fat diet and exercise regimen appears to favorably affect the levels of hormones or growth factors that influence prostate cancer growth" (*Journal of Urology* 2001; 166(3): 1185-9).

The article points out also that in Boston, an investigation that followed almost 4,000 women for 15 years found that those who had been athletes in their college days suffered 17% less breast cancer than women who had not engaged in college sports. Co-author of the study, Grace Wyshak from the Harvard School of Public Health "looked at more than 20 studies, and the weight of evidence suggests that regular physical activity does offer some protection against (breast) cancer." (*British Journal of Cancer*, 2000; 82(3): 726-30)

In these times when everyone is so busy with leisure-time activities, the National Center for Health Statistics points out that more than 30% of all men and 40% of all women report not exercising at all. The evidence from UCLA and Boston's Harvard Medical School would seem to spur both men and women in their 30's, 40's, 50's, and 60's to reprioritize their leisure-time activities. It's pretty clear that successful preventative measures are related to a combination of diet and exercise. It's only a matter of mind over matter; in light of all the evidence that's mounting, it is clear that we must *prevent* cancer or suffer the consequences!

NATIONAL CANCER INSTITUTE: Focus on Red Meat

As noted before, some of the studies that have been conducted by the National Cancer Institute have been designed to study the effects of a person's diet on risk of cancer. Recently, NCI studies show that people who ate the most red meat, averaging at least 3 ounces daily of especially well-done or fried red meats, had twice the risk of colon cancer, compared to those who ate less than half an ounce daily.

A study that NCI sponsored at the VA Medical Center in Portland, Oregon, also indicated that breast cancer risk doubled in postmenopausal women who ate 3 ounces or more of red meat a day compared with women who consumed one ounce or less daily. This study tended to confirm the results of a Vanderbilt University study that concluded that women who ate the most deep-fried, well-done, meat had nearly twice the probability of developing breast cancer as those who ate the least.

In another study conducted at the University of Minnesota, eating broiled red meat did not increase the risk of pancreatic cancer, but the odds doubled in people who ate the most grilled or barbecued red meat.

All these studies seem to say that meaty diets—particularly red meat diets like the Atkins High protein diet—*increase* the risk of cancer (but its not something you read in the Atkins Diet Books). So, if you are a "meat and potatoes" man, what should you do?

MEAT, HEAT, AND NITROSAMINES: What Science Says

According to Jean Carper (jeancarper.com), who writes and researches literature in the sciences, there are ways to sidestep cancer and (still) pack in the protein. Here's some of Carper's advice from "Eat Smart," *USA Weekend Magazine* (Jul 4–6, 2003)

1. Eat fish or poultry (and little or *no* red meat).

   In particular, Carper says that women who ate fish three or more times weekly had a 30% lower breast cancer risk than women who ate fish once a week in the VA study in Oregon. In another study (not identified by Carper), eating chicken baked, broiled or barbecued did not raise colon cancer risk, while pan-frying chicken boosted odds 50%.

2. Eat meat rare or medium rare and cook it slowly.

   At high heats (as in frying), proteins form heterocyclic amines or HCA's, which are potent carcinogens. Thus reduced heat creates fewer HCA's, with broiling produces fewer carcinogens than grilling. In the University of Minnesota study, consistently eating hamburger, beefsteak and bacon—very well done, instead of rare or medium—increased women's breast cancer risk almost five times.

3. Eat turkey or soy burgers, but not hamburgers.

   The goal is to cut down on the formation of carcinogens which are formed in the cooking process, particularly at high heat. If you mix anti-oxidants like soy protein, mashed blueberries or cherries, tea, garlic or onions into beef burger meat before cooking, Carper says you can cut the formation of carcinogens by 60% to 90%, and that reduces your risk of cancer.

4. Pre-cook meat you are going to grill.

   Since pre-cooking meat before it's grilled cuts down on the formation of those cancer-causing HCA's; pop your meat into a microwave and pre-cook it before you grill it.

5. Use "watery" sauces instead of heavy paste-sauces before grilling.

   Carper notes that some research has shown that thick tomato barbecue sauce may foster carcinogen formation. (Carper noted no research citation.)

6. Avoid nitrite-cured meats.

   Even (the late) Dr. Atkins recommended using nitrite-free bacon from healthfood stores. Most cured cold cuts, hot dogs, bacon, and ham also contain nitrites that can spur formation of nitrosamines that are known carcinogens, so, Carper notes, whenever possible, look for nitrite-free meats.

CAUTIONARY NOTES

We conclude this section on a cautionary note. The literature today on diets runs the gamut from one extreme to another. The information recently that testosterone hormone therapy (for men) is beginning to be as popular with men as hormone replacement therapy (for women) is, or was, in women. But recently, there have been side effects reported in men who used testosterone (hormone) therapy to increase their libido; there are varying opinions about unintended consequences. Doctors either like hormone replacement therapy for menopausal women or they don't like it, and there seems to be much debate with studies that support both views.

With men, testosterone (hormones)—or the diminished production of them—are thought to be the cause for everything from loss of sex drive to loss of body hair. Over the past few years, testosterone prescriptions have become increasingly popular with doctors. In 2002, almost 600,000 men age 45 and older used some form of prescription testosterone to raise the level of the sex hormone in their bodies, and the number is rising every year.

Dr. Stanley Slater is a top scientist/researcher at the National Institute on Aging (NIA), and Deputy Associate Director of NIA's geriatrics and clinical gerontology program has probably studied testosterone's effects on men longer than almost anyone else. He notes (in *Your Health*, AARP Bulletin/July-August 2003, pp 16–18) that there are safety issues to be addressed. In particular, "we know that testosterone feeds the growth of tumors in men who have metastatic prostate cancer." Thus he cautions that "most older men harbor inactive and harmless 'nests' of prostate cancer cells, and by giving extra testosterone to these men (to help their libido), we don't know if we're awakening a sleeping monster."

On the other hand, Dr. Slater doesn't specialize in prostate cancer treatment or prescribe therapies for victims of prostate cancer, so no studies have been conducted that link the use of hormone therapy with increasing levels of tumor growth (either inside or outside the prostate capsule). What we do know is that a hormone shot is administered almost immediately to the prostate cancer patient whose biopsy and body scans both indicate that the cells have migrated outside the prostate. It's still the most effective and quickest method of stopping cell growth. For that patient, the concern about the hormone's effect on increasing cell growth may be moot; if the hormone shot stops the cancer, there is no need for further study!

Just last year, however, NIH canceled a major large-scale trial after questions were raised about its design, and the director of NCI opposed it because of prostate cancer worries. It seems that scientists cannot agree on what testosterone is good for, since administering a hormone shot effectively stops cancer cells dead in their tracks. On the other hand, thousands of men are using testosterone in all different types of applications that result in renewed vigor, which makes men feel young again. For cancer victims, however, there are no scientific answers, and hormone shots remain the only high percentage method of stopping prostate cancer cells; stay tuned for further information from the scientists who continue to look for cures.

FROM THE MILKEN FOUNDATION RESEARCH

In the introduction to this primer, it was noted that the Milken Family Foundation has provided funding for prostate cancer research since the mid-1980's, totaling more than $100 million. Among its funded research projects, they have supported numerous nutrition studies and have amassed a very large data base of nutritional information. In addition to their own studies, available at their web site at www.milkenfoundation.com, they also publish numerous web sites where information can be found on general diets and nutrition.

For instance, in mid-2003 the site listed the following:

Web Site URL	Description of Information Available
www.miavita.com	This is a client-based site that provides healthy living information and nutrition ideas for employees and clients of Miavita Corporation. The info is provided free simply by going to their web site address.
www.navigator.tufts.edu	This site is maintained by nutritionists at Tufts University that provides numerous other nutrition web sites that give clear and concise information on diet and nutrition.

www.soyfoods.com	Maintained by the Indiana Soy Bean Board offers a complete directory of manufacturers of soy products like tofu and tempeh.
www.envirolinks.org.orgs.vegweb	Online guide to vegetarianism, provides more than 2000 recipes, weekly meal planners, and gardening information.
www.eatright.org/index	This is the website for the world's largest organization of dieticians with a directory of members.

Also available on the Milken Foundation site are the two cookbooks that Michael Milken (compiled by Beth Ginsberg) called *The Taste For Living World Cookbooks,* specifically for helping to fight prostate cancer. Additionally, a PDF-formatted report is available that compiles prostate-specific related nutritional information that may be helpful to sufferers with enlarged prostates as well as cancer.

All the work done by the CaP Cure research, sponsored by the Milken Foundation, is clinic-tested and has been a tremendous help in the battle to reduce prostate cancer, so men facing prostate treatment decisions must take advantage of the tremendous resources the Milken Foundation provides.

THE BEST OF THE BEST

Besides the work funded by the Milken Foundation, or should we say "including" the Milken Foundation efforts through CaP CURE, there are studies being conducted in several traditional medical settings using herbs and alternative therapies for prostate cancer. Among the top research clinics that are focused on controlled studies that use herbs in the treatment of prostate cancer is one that stands out: The Jonsson Cancer Center at the University of California-Los Angeles (UCLA).

The Jonsson Cancer Center (available on the Web at www.cancer. mednet.ucla.edu) was named by *U.S. News and World Reports* as one of the top ten cancer centers in America (Jul 21, '03 USNews.com). The rankings are charted by 150 leading physicians practicing oncology throughout more than 50 medical cancer centers in the U.S. The Jonsson Center was rated the best in California among five others that were ranked in the top 50 in the survey.

The top ten centers nationally are the M.D. Anderson Cancer Center, Houston, TX (1); Memorial Sloan-Kettering Center, New York, (2); Johns Hopkins Hospitals, Baltimore, MD, (3); Dana-Farber Cancer Institute, Boston, MA, (4); Mayo Clinic, Rochester, MN, (5); University of Chicago, Chicago, IL, (6); Duke University Medical Center, Durham, NC, (7); UCLA Jonsson Cancer, Los Angeles, CA, (8); University of Michigan Medical Center, Ann Arbor, MI, (9); and Vanderbilt University Medical Center, Nashville, TN, (10).

It should be noted that while all the cancer centers in the rankings treat prostate cancer, the Jonsson Center has a special program aimed at conducting research specifically utilizing alternative therapies and, most importantly, herbal formulations for prostate cancer. Their research is mainstream medical studies using "good scientific principles" to achieve peer-reviewed and credible scientific results. On their website they encourage interested patients to apply and become part of clinical studies, and their overall approach is aimed at learning how to reduce and/or prevent mortality from prostate cancer.

It should also be noted that the Jonsson website has links to a variety of medical journals and sources of cancer information. The herbal cancer study, either accessed through the Jonsson Center website or directly on the internet can be found at www.canceralternatives.mednet.ucla.edu and includes information on what herbs are being studied. The good news is that the mainstream medical community is beginning to integrate herbal therapies into treatment and prevention of cancer of all kinds, and it appears that the UCLA Jonsson Cancer Center is leading the effort.

Recent news from the Jonsson Cancer Center includes an announcement that for the second year in a row the doctors and prostate cancer researchers have received the largest grant of any other single institution nationwide. A grant totaling $1 million was awarded by CaP CURE, the Michael Milken Foundation that is profiled elsewhere in this text. Dr. Charles Sawyers, head of the Prostate Cancer Center at the Jonsson Center, noted that

> (The combined research at the Center) "…has been providing new insights into molecular disease mechanisms (represented in prostate cancer) and targeted organs such as breast cancer, leukemia, and lymphoma and its easy to envision how these same strategies might be brought to bear on prostate cancer (with the new monies provided by CaP Cure added to existing funding.)"

The herbal studies program, announced in January, 2003, was funded with $1.1 million and is being carried out at the Sue Stiles Program in Integrative Oncology, and according to a news release (www.nbc4tv.health), will focus on

> "…an untapped goldmine of plant life and natural compounds that haven't been tested as potential cancer fighters….such things as components of shark liver oil, soy and yerba santa, a plant historically used by Native Americans for healing."

In a comment by the Director of Integrative Oncology at the Jonsson Center, Dr. Richard Pietras noted that

> "These plants and compounds could one day replace more toxic and debilitating chemotherapies now in use…I hope that we will one day be able to *treat cancer* patients with less harmful and more targeted therapies to fight their tumors and relieve their symptoms."

Dr. Pietras also noted that

> "…of the 92 drugs approved for cancer treatment from 1983 to 1994, 62 were derived from natural sources and…more than 50 Million compounds have never been screened for tumor-fighting properties (in controlled studies)."

It is encouraging that the mainstream medical community is recognizing the importance of herbs and supplements as valid medical prescription alternatives.

6

Exciting New Therapies for Prostate Cancer

In this chapter you will learn about...

FUTURE TREATMENTS: Cryogenics, Vaccines, Robot-Assisted RP....

PHOTODYNAMIC THERAPY

Turn Up the Heat

SNAKE OIL: BEWARE!

GOOD NEWS FOR PROSTATECTAMIES (And Other Treatments, Too!)

FINASTERIDE TRIALS: The Latest Results

Upside versus Downside: You Decide

INTRODUCTION

Researchers at University College London Hospital in England have been treating many types of cancer, including prostate cancer, with a method they have labeled "photodynamic therapy" (PDT). At the London hospital, they used the therapy on 14 men whose prostate cancer had come back after being treated with radiation. First the patients got an intravenous injection of the photosensitive drug, then they waited three days for the drug to migrate into the tumor(s). At that point, the doctors shined (laser) light on the tumors to activate the photosensitive drug, which destroys the tumors.

It is still in the development stages, but researchers believe PDT will have few complications or side-effects, once the therapy is perfected. So it appears this therapy not only has great promise for the patient who has previously been treated for cancer of the prostate, but also as a possible treatment for newly discovered prostate cancer which is contained within the capsule.

Many more trials and more research remains to be done, but this is probably one of the highest probability therapies with the greatest promise for prostate cancer treatment that is being studied at the present time.

TURN UP THE HEAT

There is an interesting internet web site that features a Naturopathic Physician answering questions about alternative medicine and treatments for all kinds of maladies, including cancer. In a recent issue of www.letstalkhealth.com (Volume 5, Number 3 Newsletter), editor Kurt W. Donsbach discussed the use of an old treatment called Delwa-Star H & P thermo-therapy for treating hemorrhoids. Dr. Donsbach noted also that recently he had seen dramatic results when the "device" was used for prostatic hypertrophy. The thermotherapy is based on the concept that an increase in temperature of the tissue produces an irrigation of blood to the area concerned and relaxes the musculature around it, allowing an even greater flow. Dr. Donsbach notes that when the thermotheraputic probe was applied for consecutive periods of time, there was an observed reduction in the prostate (size) and "actually reverses itself, thereby relieving symptoms (of BPH) and side effects."

Donsbach indicated that "the concept is proven now for both hemorrhoids and prostatic conditions," although he does not cite any specific studies supporting his thesis. It is unclear whether or not any studies have been done on the use of thermotheraputic probes for prostate cancer, but in most men over the age of 70, cancer is almost always preceded by lengthy problems with BPH. Thus it is possible that shrinking the gland by thermotheraputic applications may slow, or even eliminate, the onset of cancer in the gland. Again, no studies are cited and none have been found in the literature, although several cancer clinics indicated that they are experimenting with thermo-treatment applications for prostate cancer.

SNAKE OIL: Beware!

In medicine, cures for every malady known to man (and woman) have been touted for centuries throughout history by charlatans of every kind. Most "remedies" turned out to be shams to make the morbidity of the general public a cash cow for the purveyors. Today, with the tremendous growth of the World Wide Web (Internet) just in this new millennium, literally thousands of web sites are touting cancer cures that rival all the snake oil salesmen that ever plied their trade.

Recently, the AARP surfed the Internet to see what's being "sold" as sure-fire cancer cures, and they were amazed to learn that "what's eluded the world's leading medical researchers around the globe is already available, and in more than one "clinical" setting: a cure for cancer!" (*AARP Journal*, January 2003).

There are "cures" that are available from both women and men who've found *the answer* (to various cancer-types, including prostate cancer) for the low, low price of $18.95, and there are cures that use everything from powdered shark cartilage to hydrazine sulfate that are "guaranteed" to eradicate cancer—almost overnight! Some cancer products and therapy sites sell videos that promise—much like the circus barkers—that cancer will virtually "leap right out of the body," right before your very eyes!

Just in case you are tempted to spend your money, you probably should check with other authorities, like the FTC, before you send in a check. The Bulletin also notes that a good place to learn about cancer quackery is right on the internet, available at www.quackwatch.org.

All this is not to say there isn't good information, or perhaps, even remedies for prostate cancer that have no clinical trials or history, yet which are being looked at by very good research clinics. There are many great hospitals and clinics that have web sites, some that have been referenced in this book, so the message is: be cautious when conducting your research on the Internet. It's a whole new world of possibilities, and you deserve not to be scammed.

In the final analysis, if you have been diagnosed with prostate cancer, use any and all means of getting good information about your options. And good health and a long life is our wish for you!

GOOD NEWS FOR PROSTATECTOMIES

It was mentioned in Chapter Two that robotics have been introduced into the Retropubic Prostatectomy surgery procedures just in the recent two or three years (since about 2000). And while it is not our intent to endorse a particular clinic, or even to recommend a particular procedure for prostate cancer, it is certainly important that we provide you with options, and from our research, names of doctors who have the most experience in any of these procedures.

In the late 1990's, the da Vinci laparoscopic (robotic) radical prostatectomy procedure was being pioneered and performed in France. Through the late '90's, clinics in the U.S. and Europe acquired the equipment and began to train surgeons on this precision process for removing the prostate gland. What they learned, through several hundred robot-assisted radical prostatectomies, was that this new robotic technique had a better result when compared with the historical non-robotic surgery procedures then (and now) in more common practice.

Reports in the *Journal of Urology* (Vol. 163, 2000) by Guillonneau and Vallancien and in 2001, (Vol. 165) peaked interest in the radical prostatectomy/urology community, and clinics from Los Angeles to New York began training and using the method as an alternative to traditional open anatomic RP. One of the first clinics to embrace the da Vinci technique was the Vattikuti Institute at Henry Ford Health Systems in Detroit, Michigan.

The Vatti Institute has developed a reputation as a leader in successful robotic-assisted prostatectomies that is rivaled by few other U.S. prostate cancer specialists. Their success, while still too infant to know longevity statistics (i.e. they have been perfoming da Vinci prostatectomies only since 2001), has been reported in papers by the head of their team, which includes Dr. Mani Menon, Ashutosh Tewari, and James Peabody (and their VIP Team members) in the *Journal of Urology* in both November 2002 and June of 2003. "Success," in the case of the Vatti Institute, is measured in comparison with traditional open anatomic RP's in the following ways:

> **"Results: In the last 100 cases, mean operative time was 2.5 hours with average blood loss of 150 ml. Median specimen Gleason score was 7 and mean tumor volume was 7 cc....patients were discharged on average, in less than 24 hours and mean catherterization time was 4.2 days. Conclu-**

sion: The Vattikuti Institute prostatectomy is a precise and safe minimally invasive technique of radical retropubic prostatectomy…"

(M. Menon; et al, *Journal of Urology*, June 2003).

When compared with traditional (non-robotic) retropubic RP's, average blood loss is two to three times more than the robot-assisted procedure, hospital duration is 4 to 5 days, catheter duration is measured in weeks, and pain significantly more acute (as reported by retrospective follow-up) for traditional surgery patients. (M. Menon; et al, *Journal of Urology,* Nov 2002).

But all is not positive yet; there are some downsides to robotic-assisted RP. The first note (by the authors, Menon, et al) is a cautionary one: Not enough patients have been treated with the da Vinci procedure to draw inferences at this point in time. Therefore, as more procedures are accomplished and more statistics are quantified and published, this could become the gold standard of prostatectomy procedures (as the non-robotic laparoscopic procedure is now).

The biggest problem with the da Vinci procedure is cost. In 2002, the Vitti Institute reported that typical cost of the robot-assisted procedure was approaching $1 million, and insurance companies were not covering it because the data was not yet developed to show it was worth that much. In addition, the costs of equipment and recurring cost of consumables are almost prohibitive. The procedure takes at least 3 surgeons—not counting the one handling the robotic controls—plus support staff that are highly specialized in the procedure.

Over time, however, those costs will decline and skilled personnel will be trained and available. Consumables and associated operating room costs will decline also. The time in the hospital will, in some measures, offset follow-up care-costs, and the associated support staff and consumables will do the same. Thus by the time this information is in print, costs may not be such an impediment, although rising health care costs now being borne by the consumer is increasing at the rate of 15% a year, so it remains to be seen.

One thing is certain: The Vitti Institute will be at the forefront of Robotic Radical Retropubic Prostatectomy research and the prostate cancer victim should explore this option if surgery is suggested. It most assuredly is the gold standard for the way prostatectamies will be performed in the future.

AFTER A PROSTATECTOMY: What If?

Let's just think about the unthinkable: what if a prostatectomy has been performed and has resulted in the dreaded "erectile dysfunction" (ED). What's the prognosis for a cure?

Recently, there have been studies using Viagra (sildenafil) for prostate cancer patients after treatment. Reuters Health (New York, April, 2003) studied men for nine months after having their prostates removed and found some interesting results. The study was conducted by Dr. Harin Padma-Nathan of the University of Southern California in LA, where they asked 23 and 28 men to take 50 milligrams and 100 milligrams of Viagra, respectively, every night for nine months, starting four weeks after the radical prostatectomy. Another 25 men took a placebo during the same time period. None of the men knew whether they were taking Viagra or a placebo, and all of the men had normal erectile function before surgery.

Padma-Nathan discovered that 27 % of men who had received Viagra, regardless of dose (some were given 100 mls and some were given 50 mls), had regained full erectile functioning equal to what they reported before undergoing surgery, while only 4% of the men given the placebo recovered erectile function.

No serious side effects were reported by any of the Viagra group and Padma-Nathan concluded that "doing nothing is not good. Intervention (i.e. using Viagra) certainly made it a whole lot better."

Given that the men in the study were in their mid-50's, it means there is hope for resumption of a normal sex life after prostate surgery, although there is an expense associated with Viagra. On the other hand, Padma-Nathan noted that animal studies have shown that the drug may actually be restoring or reattaching nerves that are damaged in the surgery, thereby giving hope that the medication may actually "fix" the problem and erectile function might return without intervention later on. Of course it's too soon to tell if that's possible, but there's hope.

The good news is that use of sildenfil for prostate cancer treated with other means, like brachytherapy or E-Beam, can provide even stronger erections, especially in the early months following treatment. And it is yet another opportunity to show that the medical community is moving forward in prostate cancer *recovery* research, even as new cancer elimination treatments are being found.

FINASTERIDE TRIALS

If you have been watching national news lately, you probably are already aware of the trials conducted under the direction of the National Cancer Institute and published in the June 2003 issue of the *New England Journal of Medicine*. The study utilized the BPH-reduction drug, "finasteride," in a study at University of Texas Health Sciences Center in San Antonio, where 18,000 men over the age of 60 were tracked for more than seven years.

The most popular use for finasteride—or Proscar, as it is named on the prescription market—although in significantly less dosage than was administered in this study is for baldness prevention. It is also used for BPH sufferers, and the study utilized similar dosage in this study as that used for the purpose of reducing the symptoms of prostate gland enlargement.

Dr. Ian Thompson was the principle investigator on the study, and he noted that Proscar alters levels of the male hormone, DHT, a testosterone relative. It has already been determined that men with naturally low levels of DHT have less prostate cancer, and that Black (American) men who generally have a very high risk of prostate cancer have high DHT levels, also. In this study, researchers tested whether reducing DHT could prevent cancer, and what they found was that men who took the drug every day for seven years reduced the risk of prostate cancer by 25 percent (15 fewer cancers in 1,000 men), as measured against the men in the study who were administered a placebo over the same period.

UPSIDE vs. DOWNSIDE

While the news that prostate cancer might be prevented and there might someday be a pill that every man could take to drive the risk of having cancer later on, appears to be supported by the results of this study, there are some downside cautions to consider. The doctors conducting the study noted that Proscar can cause sexual "problems," and although not confirmed precisely by the study, the percentage of those men who did have prostate cancer during the study appeared to have slightly more aggressive tumors than would have been expected in the normal population.

It should be noted that men in this study had biopsies of their prostate glands, regardless of what their PSA levels were, in order to confirm tumors were present. Interestingly, researchers diagnosed prostate cancer in four times more placebo patients than expected in the normal population (non-trial-participants). Most tumors discovered were small, early-stage tumors, which would not have triggered a biopsy under normal examination conditions.

The fact that the rate was four times higher than expected in the placebo group is actually consistent with the study noted earlier in this text (Chapter Two) where the autopsies showed a very high presence of cancer tumors in prostates of men of all ages. But this study's researchers made no comment about the significance of the findings in that regard.

What they did conclude is that the study gives hope that one day a vaccine or pill may be found that will be able to reduce prostate cancer, much like the polio and small pox vaccines have accomplished for those diseases. Right now, however, they caution that the upside and downside of Finasteride therapy needs to be weighed by each individual who contemplates using it in the hope of preventing prostate cancer from occurring. Since the study didn't test whether taking the drug helped men live longer, American Cancer Society's Dr. Herman Kattlove predicted that there will be a huge debate about its usefulness.

Suffice it to say, for our purposes in providing men of all ages with information about prostate cancer, this study is yet another positive indication that eventually it may be possible to have a pill that can be taken early on to prevent the onset of cancer that is the second leading cancer that causes men to die today.

PARTING SHOTS

It has been said in other parts of this book that because men are the way they are, almost anything of a medical nature that affects areas "below the belt" and above the knees, is ginger territory. Women, on the other hand, because of their very biological differences, seem to be more at ease in dealing with problems in those areas of their bodies.

Men also are used to hearing all the jokes and, over the years of growing into a fully functional sexual animal, have seen and heard all the penis jokes and urban legends. Believe it or not, many men also still believe in the adage that "bigger is better" when it comes to penis size, although women, at least when asked if that would be their personal belief, would be mostly reluctant to endorse such statements.

The literature is vague on this as it relates to prostate cancer treatment(s), but in discussions with both doctors who perform radical prostatectamies and with men who have had that surgery, it is fairly common knowledge that erections (post-operative) result in shorter penis length by one to 1 ½ inches, on average (based on those self-descriptions).

For brachytherapy, there appears to also be a reduction in length, but perhaps less than half an inch, although the rigidity of the erection seems to be diminished somewhat from before the implant procedure was performed. But it still performs as before, and most men say they've had no complaints.

The literature is silent on both these issues, but the anecdotal evidence is fairly consistent. So, should that impact a man's decision (or a couple) on which treatment to choose? Of course not! But it is an issue you won't find discussed anywhere else, at least not in popular literature dealing with prostate cancer.

Now you have the tools necessary to make good decisions. Your prostate health and your future is in your hands now, and I am confident the decisions you will make will ensure a long and healthy life. Thank you for choosing this little *primer* for helping you with your decision-making process.

FINAL NOTES: Don't Take Newspaper Accounts As Gospel

Every time someone "famous" learns they have prostate cancer or divulges to the press that they will be treated for prostate cancer, the newspapers bring the disease into the public's view once more. Recent examples include former New York City mayor, Rudy Gulliani; Senator (and Presidential-wannabe) John Kerry; and Secretary of State Colin Powell.

Always accompanying those press announcements is a brief discussion of the "treatment" that the individual chose and a review of statistics of the disease, but the information is almost always summarized in a manner that downplays the seriousness with which choice of treatment should be addressed. For instance, in both Kerry and Powell's cases the press reported that "surgery would result in a complete cure and they would be back on the political treadmill in a matter of days with no noticeable after-effects…"

In Powell's case, articles appeared on the same (newspaper) that described what a prostatectomy involves and quoted statistics that separated men by age into categories. Seventy-five percent of those men over age 70 will have sexual dysfunction (no erection capability), while only one-third of those men under 50 who have their prostate gland removed will lose sexual capability! No word on the men between 50 and 70 years of age who choose radical prostatectomy, yet that's the largest age group diagnosed!

In addition, the press seems to extol the virtues of surgery for men who detect the disease in the early stages (i.e. before there is evidence it has spread outside the gland) on the basis that lympth nodes in the groin area can be removed at the same time during the prostatectomy and tested. It is presented very subtly, but for the uneducated and uninformed reader, the implication is (once again!) that getting the organ removed guarantees the cure!

By now, if you have been paying attention throughout this primer, you have learned to read between the lines about any and all things medical. And once again, it is clear that news from our media should reinforce the two messages that this primer is hoping to make clear:

1. Younger and younger men are being diagnosed with prostate cancer, so beginning the PSA and DRE screening needs to occur at age 45 or earlier for men who have a family history;

2. A positive diagnosis means it is time to start researching treatment options—including obtaining second and third opinions from urologists, brachytherapists, and other medical professionals who specialize in prostate cancer.

APPENDIX

Some Other References…

Khalsa, Dharma Singh, *Meditation As Medicine*, Pocket Books, New York, NY, 2001

__, April 19, 02; "Tomatoes cut prostate cancer risk", *Arizona Republic* (AP Release)

Advertising Supplement, May 2, '02; Cancer Research, et al.; *Arizona Republic* (SF Examiner)

__, May 9, 02, "Cancer link to vaccine discovered"; *Arizona Republic*

__, March 5, 2002; "Blood test for breast cancer sought"; *Arizona Republic* (AP Release)

__, AP; May 21, 2002, *Arizona Republic*; pg A5

Carper, Jean, (1997); *Miracle Cures*, Harper-Collins, NY, NY

NCCN, www.national comprehensive cancer…; 2001

__, April, '02, Vol 3, #2, "Quercetin May Be A Natural Treatment for Prostate Cancer"; *Healthkeepers* Magazine

Mattern, H., May 5, '02, "The world as Herb sees it"; *Arizona Republic*

O'Hara, M.; (2001); *Prostate Cancer Battle: It's Strictly Your Decision*, 1st Books Online (at 1stbooks.com)

__. www.MayoClinic.com; 2001–2002

__, July, 2001; *Your Prostate Health* (Newsletter), Grado—Ragde Clinics, (distributed sporadically throughout the year to the medical community)

Goodman, Jack M., (1997),"Prostate Cancer: Some Things Every Man Should Know" (Brochure), Available from VIVUS, Inc, 4469 W. Avalon, Phoenix, AZ 85031

Sheldon, S; Cedars Sinia Hospital (personal interview), April, 2001

The Healthy Cell News, Spring 2002, "You Can Prevent and Even Stop Prostate Problems," ALV Publishers, Inc., PO Box 250, Young, AZ 85554

AARP Bulletin/January 2003; July/Aug 2003; (www.aarp.org/bulletin)

More References....

Clapp, Larry; *Prostate Health in 90 Days,* 9th printing-Feb. '99, Hay House, Inc., Carlsbad, CA.

Schachter, Michael, M.D., www.World Health OnLine (2001–2002)

"Prostate: For Men and Women Who Care About Them"; *Today's Arizona Woman,* June 2002

Bostwick, D., MacLennan, G., and Larson, T*.; Prostate Cancer-What Every Man—And His Family—Should Know;* 1996, (American Cancer Society); Random House, Inc.; NY, NY

US News & World Report, "Cancer: New Promise For Early Detection", Vol 132, No. 22, June 24, 2002, pp 48–58

National Prostate Cancer Council (NPCC.com); June 2002

Hsing, Ann W., *Journal of the National Cancer Institute*, (*Arizona Republic*, October 15, 2002

Evans, Mark, "Gene Tied to Deadly Prostate Cancer," October 9, 2002, AP Wire Story; http://apnews.excite.com/article/20021009/D7MI76EO0.html

(www.letstalkhealth.com); Newsletter (Vol 5, #3: Oct/Nov 2002); 1229 3rd Ave, Ste. C; Chula Vista, CA 91911

www.Yahoo! News—Viagra; Reuter News Limited, (Accessed) April 28, 2003

New England Journal of Medicine, I. Thompson, PI, June, 2003

Carper, J., "Eat Smart, High-Protein Hazards"; *USA Weekend Magazine* (usaweekend.com); Jul 4–6, 2003; pp 4.

Wentworth, R., (2002), *Caught With My Pants Down*, 1st Books Online at 1stbooks.com

__ JonssonCenter.com; (Aug03)"Update on Herbal and Alternative Medicine Research," (Internet Web Site for UCLA Cancer Research Center); Fall 2003

bostwicklaboratories.com; 2004-glossary/definitions

About the Author

Nicholas R. Hild has been a Professor and researcher at Arizona State University for more than 20 years. While he has focused his work in the environmental health and safety field, his recent diagnosis and subsequent treatment for Prostate Cancer led to this seminal work being published. Dr. Hild noted that, "my work in the field of environmental health was invaluable in learning about the issues that face 300,000 men each year who receive the dreaded news that they have Prostate Cancer. The journey I took to find the best available treatment made it imperative that I share the many sources of prostate options with doctors, clinics, and diagnosed men everywhere, to help with this insidious disease."

Dr. Hild is a Professor of Environmental Technology Management at Arizona State University, where he resides in the desert splendor of rural Pinal County.

0-595-31125-3

www.ingramcontent.com/pod-product-compliance
Lightning Source LLC
Chambersburg PA
CBHW030859180526
45163CB00004B/1638